D0496682

Evaluation

Jackie Green and Jane South

Open University Press

Open University Press
McGraw-Hill Education
McGraw-Hill House
Shoppenhangers Road
Maidenhead
Berkshire
England
SL6 2QL

email: enquiries@openup.co.uk
world wide web: www.openup.co.uk

and Two Penn Plaza, New York, NY 10121-2289, USA

First published 2006

Copyright © Jackie Green and Jane South 2006

All rights reserved. Except for the quotation of short passages for the purpose of criticism and review, no part of this publication may be reproduced, stored in a retrieval system, or transmitted, in any form or by any means, electronic, mechanical, photocopying, recording or otherwise, without the prior written permission of the publisher or a licence from the Copyright Licensing Agency Limited. Details of such licences (for reprographic reproduction) may be obtained from the Copyright Licensing Agency Ltd of 90 Tottenham Court Road, London W1T 4LP.

A catalogue record of this book is available from the British Library

ISBN-10: 0 335 21915 2 (pb) 0 335 21916 0 (hb)
ISBN-13: 978 0 335 21915 5 (pb) 978 0 335 21916 2 (hb)

Library of Congress Cataloging-in-Publication Data
CIP data applied for

Typeset by RefineCatch Limited, Bungay, Suffolk
Printed in Poland by OZGraf. S.A.
www.polskabook.pl

Edge Hill University
Learning Services

Barcode 296 770

Contents

Preface to the series

The current public health and social policy context is rapidly changing. Current policy initiatives resound with terms such as community engagement, social inclusion, equity, participation, empowerment and evidence-based practice. Responsibility for delivering the agenda ultimately resides with the public health workforce and puts pressure on practitioners to embrace new methods and ways of working. There is also unprecedented pressure to evaluate work and demonstrate achievement of targets.

Our experience of working with practitioners and those training for practice is that while they grasp the significance of many of these new ideas and ways of working, they often feel ill-prepared to translate the rhetoric into meaningful activity on the ground. This series of texts, *Key Concepts for Public Health Practice*, will take some of the most significant issues in the emerging wider public health agenda and attempt to 'unlock the maze'. Rather than providing a simple 'how to' guide, the series will offer clear, accessible explanations of the core principles and theory which readers will be able to apply across different contexts and for a range of purposes. Because nothing is as simple as it seems, it will also provide insights into dealing with some of the 'real-life' challenges and complexities of contemporary UK practice.

Each volume in the series will address a major contemporary issue. All the volumes will conform to a common format. Section A will provide an overview of relevant theory and will draw out key concepts and principles. Section B will demonstrate how these principles can be applied in practice using illustrative examples and case studies. Section C will provide an honest discussion of some of the thorny issues and dilemmas arising in 'real-life' practice.

Acknowledgements

Our thinking about evaluation and our ideas for this book have been shaped by the many people we have worked with on evaluation projects. In particular, we would like to thank the following individuals for allowing us to use their work as illustrative examples – Pat Fairfax, Eleanor Green, Hawarun Hussain, Jill Kibble, Liz Murray, Caroline Newell, Alyson Nicholds, Jill Salvin and Alan White.

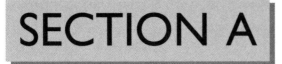

SECTION A

Principles

1 | Introduction – setting the scene

Overview

This chapter provides an introduction to the book and, in particular, focuses on:

- the purpose of evaluation
- the scope of modern public health
- internal and external evaluation
- commissioning evaluation.

The pressure to evaluate

Some years ago Pawson and Tilley (1997: 1) likened evaluation to 'a vast lumbering overgrown adolescent. . . . It does not know quite where it is going and it is prone to bouts of despair'. Whether it has matured into a sophisticated adult during the intervening years is debatable. However, it is undeniable that it has become much more pervasive and, some might feel, intrusive. Whereas in the past evaluation tended to be confined to major programmes and so-called demonstration projects, it is now part and parcel of everyday professional activity. In both the public and voluntary sectors, the receipt of funding, for even small-scale projects, carries with it the obligation to evaluate. Notwithstanding the increased pressure to evaluate, it is our experience that for many people working within the wider field of public health, evaluation is not their main priority and may even be seen as taking up valuable time and resources that could be better spent on improving health.

↻ Points for reflection

Reflect on your own views about evaluation by completing the following sentence stems.

At worst evaluation can be . . .

At best evaluation can be . . .

The purpose of this volume is to demonstrate that evaluation is integral to good practice and to establish key principles which will assist in carrying out, commissioning or interpreting evaluation. In short, it aims to enable the reader to maximize the positive aspects of evaluation and minimize the negative. To this end, Section A will provide a pathway through the theory and principles of evaluation and Section B will show how these can be applied in practice. Section C, with due deference to Murphy's Law that nothing is as simple as it seems, will tackle some of the more contentious or challenging aspects of evaluation.

Why evaluate?

At its most basic, evaluation is concerned with assessing whether interventions are effective. There is considerable debate about how effectiveness and success are judged. Clearly, different stakeholders will hold different views stemming from their different aspirations for an intervention and, indeed, what type of evidence they find convincing. Notwithstanding these differences, which will be discussed more fully in Chapter 2, justifications for funding and obtaining renewal of funding are frequently dependent on evidence of success. The increasing emphasis on such evidence has been associated with 'economic rationalism' and the need to ensure that public funds are being used to best effect (Raphael 2000). However, for many the primary concern is not with accountability, but with what can be learned from the experience of implementing initiatives. The World Health Organization (WHO 1998: 3) refers to the role of evaluation in capacity building and enhancing the ability of 'individuals, communities, organizations and governments to address important health concerns'.

Clearly, establishing whether interventions 'have worked' – or equally 'have not worked' – is integral to evidence-based practice and of potential interest to the wider public health workforce. Such evidence can be used to inform future developments from local projects through to major policy change. However, wider dissemination and implementation will prove to be problematic unless there is some complementary understanding of the factors associated with success or failure. As Feuerstein (1986: 7) contends, 'Knowing *why* a programme succeeds or fails is even more important than knowing that it does'.

Evaluation has long been recognized as fundamental to good practice and to be a core component of the health promotion planning cycle as shown in Figure 1.1. From the perspective of those more directly involved with initiatives being evaluated, the findings can be used to review progress and make any necessary amendments to keep the project on track. Equally, demonstrating achievement and celebrating success can provide further motivation and empower individuals (Springett 1998a). Barr *et al.* (1996) make the point that evaluation can check whether the benefits of action to promote health are equitably distributed and reach those most in need. This is clearly important if efforts to promote health are to contribute to a reduction in health inequalities. Chapter 7 will focus on how to involve hard-to-reach groups in evaluation.

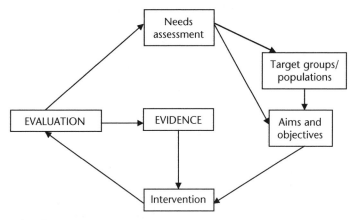

Figure 1.1 The health promotion planning cycle

Evaluation also has a major role in protecting the public from inappropriate or harmful practices. Clearly, there is an ethical obligation to ensure that interventions do no harm, either indirectly by squandering limited resources on ineffective interventions or, indeed, more directly. Ineffective and inappropriate interventions may alienate community groups and make them more resistant to other attempts to bring about change. Further, even well-intentioned and apparently plausible programmes may be harmful. A useful illustration is provided by the former practice of putting babies to sleep on their side, which appeared to make sense as it resembled the recovery position. However, this practice was subsequently shown to be associated with increased risk of sudden infant death syndrome and replaced by the 'back to sleep' message. There is a further obligation to ensure that the way evaluation is conducted conforms with ethical principles. These issues will be discussed more fully in Chapter 6.

Those involved in commissioning or carrying out evaluations may have different purposes in mind. Lewis (2001: 392) notes the high regard in which evaluation for accountability is currently held and calls for a 'campaign for more evaluation for learning – of both process and impact'. We might distinguish four primary purposes for evaluation:

- evaluation for accountability
- evaluation for learning
- evaluation for programme management and development
- evaluation as an ethical obligation.

What is being evaluated – the nature of modern public health

Although the principles of evaluation are applicable within a number of fields, the emphasis in this text is on the modern, multidisciplinary public health as envisaged in the white paper *Saving Lives: Our Healthier Nation* (Department of Health 1999), the *Report of the Chief Medical Officer's Project to Strengthen the Public Health Function* in England (Chief Medical Officer 2001) and *Shifting the Balance of Power* (Department of Health 2001b). It includes three major groups of staff as identified in the earlier Chief Medical Officer's project on strengthening the public health workforce (Department of Health 1998):

- public health specialists
- public health practitioners
- the wider workforce including the voluntary sector.

Health Promotion plays a key role and has been at the forefront of debates about evaluation methodology and the development of approaches which are both robust and consistent with values and ways of working. These arguments will feature prominently in this text, and it is therefore appropriate to briefly consider the position of Health Promotion *vis-à-vis* Public Health. (Note that we use 'Public Health' to refer to the 'profession' as opposed to 'public health' to refer to the wide grouping of different professions and organizations involved in activity to improve health.) Tilford *et al.* (2003) have explored the origin of Health Promotion in the 1980s as a response to:

- acknowledgement of the holistic nature of health
- appreciation of the limitations of high-tech medicine in improving the health status of populations
- recognition of the broad determinants of health and particularly the impact of environmental factors
- criticism of attempts to manipulate behaviour through educational approaches which overlooked environmental constraints on behaviour and the absence of free choice – generally associated with the notion of victim blaming (Ryan 1976; Rodmell and Watt 1986).

Historically, as Health Promotion sought to establish itself as a discipline and a profession, it struggled to distance itself from Public Health and particularly the medical model which dominated twentieth-century thinking about health. It took a holistic view of health incorporating positive well-being rather than focusing on disease. It challenged the emphasis on individual behaviour and addressed the 'upstream' wider determinants of health. A WHO Working Group on Health Promotion Evaluation listed the basic principles that characterize the 'health promotion' way of working. These are listed in Box 1.1.

The origins of Public Health as a discipline can be traced to the nineteenth-century increase in awareness of the environmental causes of disease and the

Box 1.1 Core principles of health promotion

Health promotion is:

- empowering (enabling individuals and communities to assume more power over the personal, socio-economic and environmental factors that affect their health)
- participatory (involving all concerned at all stages of the process)
- holistic (fostering physical, mental, social and spiritual health)
- intersectoral (involving the collaboration of agencies from relevant sectors)
- equitable (guided by a concern for equity and social justice)
- sustainable (bringing about changes that individuals and communities can maintain once initial funding has ended)
- multi-strategy (using a variety of approaches – including policy development, organizational change, community development, legislation, advocacy, education and communication – in combination) (Rootman *et al.* 2001: 4–5).

sanitary reform movement. Developments in biomedicine and a focus on micro-causality progressively shifted the emphasis towards personal prevention and individual lifestyles and behaviours. The emergence of the 'New Public Health' in the late twentieth century was an attempt to move away from this emphasis on individual responsibility for health towards consideration of the social, economic and environmental factors that collectively influence health and health action. In many ways this could be seen as reconciling Health Promotion with Public Health. However, critics have asserted that despite the rhetoric, the New Public Health has not freed itself from concern with individual responsibility for health (Petersen and Lupton 1996). Tilford *et al.*'s (2003) analysis of the values in Health Promotion and Public Health noted some differences. In relation to the relative emphasis on terminal values (ends) or instrumental values (means), Public Health tended to have a greater emphasis on ends whereas for Health Promotion it was the means of achieving them. Terminal values common to both were equity, equality, justice, autonomy, empowerment, but prevention and protection also featured as terminal values for Public Health. Health Promotion, in contrast, was held to have a more holistic view of health and a stronger emphasis on processes around involvement, participation, autonomy and contributing to empowerment. Notwithstanding these differences, the emergence of the modern multidisciplinary public health provides an umbrella term for bringing together all those whose work might positively impact on the health of communities and populations. However, awareness of alternative value positions may be helpful in interpreting some of the debates about evaluation which have centred on the definition of goals, the relative emphasis on process or outcomes and the ways in which these should be measured. These debates form a thread throughout this book.

The scope of public health practice

The Ottawa Charter (WHO 1986) established guiding principles for Health Promotion and remains a key point of reference for those working in both Health Promotion and Public Health. It identified five key action areas:

- building healthy public policy
- creating supportive environments
- strengthening community action
- developing personal skills
- reorienting health services.

The range of initiatives to improve health is clearly very wide-ranging in scope, approach and content. It includes major policy development on specific health issues such as tobacco policy, as well as more 'upstream' determinants such as economic or housing policy. It also encompasses more discrete small-scale projects such as setting up a food co-operative or providing a parenting course for teenage mothers. However, the emphasis is on social rather than biomedical or clinical interventions. The focus is on population groups of varying size, from whole populations to small community groups, rather than on individuals. We use the terms 'intervention', 'initiative', 'programme' or 'project' to refer to any aspect of the whole spectrum of activity that characterizes the 'wider' public health. There is a clear distinction, then, between individually orientated biomedical interventions and broader public health interventions that are more complex both in themselves and in the range of possible outcomes they achieve.

Parry-Langdon *et al.* (2003) suggest that anticipated outcomes in health promotion are often poorly defined, and valued outcomes such as empowerment and participation are difficult to measure. To address this complexity, Nutbeam (1998: 41) issues four key challenges which emerge from his analysis of evaluation. These are:

- using research evidence more systematically in the planning of activities
- improving the definition and measurement of outcome
- adopting appropriate evaluation intensity
- adopting appropriate evaluation design.

We respond to these challenges by unpacking the principles of evaluation, examining design and measurement issues in the context of real practice and considering how evaluation findings can be used to best effect.

Who evaluates?

Tones and Tilford (1994: 49) note that the early literature on the evaluation of social programmes tends to be concerned with evaluation as an 'independent and external element'. More recently, however, evaluation has become more integrated within programme delivery and is more likely to involve practitioners themselves. The decision whether or not to commission an external evaluator may ultimately depend on the resources available. However, the 'hidden' costs of using internal staff should not be overlooked. WHO (1998) recommends that at least 10 per cent of the project budget should be used for evaluation. Over and above any financial considerations, there are a number of issues related to the overall purpose of the evaluation, which may influence the choice between external and internal evaluator. As external evaluators are independent of the project, they are often seen as objective and impartial. They can bring specialist expertise and a fresh eye to interpreting situations. They may therefore become aware of issues which those more closely involved have become inured to. Their independence of management and other power structures may make it easier for people to speak frankly and also to produce an independent report. However, because of their role, external evaluators may also be seen as intimidating by project staff, whatever their personal qualities and style of working. It is essential that trust and good working relationships are established so that staff are aware of the positive benefits of evaluation, are willing to co-operate and feel able to communicate freely.

Alternatively, people who are directly involved in delivering the project or intervention can be used as internal evaluators. Internal evaluators may have a vested interest in the project and risk being less objective than external evaluators – or at least being seen to be so. They may also have less experience in evaluation and their reports may carry less 'authority' than those of external evaluators. However, internal evaluators may have more insight into the project itself and the context within which it is being provided, and this familiarity can assist in interpreting what is happening. Involvement in evaluation also helps to establish ownership of the findings and engender greater willingness to make any required changes to practice.

It is not uncommon for external evaluators to work collaboratively with internal evaluators in a variety of ways, including the development and co-ordination of an evaluation strategy and training of internal evaluators. The success of such an approach depends on agreeing respective roles and responsibilities. However, it can be argued that such collaboration capitalizes on the strengths of both types of evaluator (Katz and Peberdy 1997).

Critics such as Feuerstein (1986) have challenged the use of expert-led evaluation for community-based projects. Members of the community and community workers are required to provide information but have little if any say about what the evaluation focuses on, the form it takes and any decisions taken on the basis of the findings. She refers to it as the 'studying the specimens' type of evaluation. In contrast, the 'real partnership in development' type of evaluation involves the community at every stage of the process. WHO (1998) suggests that those with a legitimate interest in an initiative should be involved at each stage of the evaluation. This includes policymakers, members of the community, organizations, health and other professionals, local and national health agencies. WHO further recommends that the adoption of participatory approaches to evaluation should be encouraged. The use of participatory and collaborative approaches will be discussed more fully in Chapters 5 and 6.

Commissioning evaluation

Successful commissioning is clearly dependent on achieving a good fit between the purpose and scope of the evaluation and the capability of those tendering. In many instances there will be a formal tendering process which will require precise specification of the aims of the evaluation, time-scales and constraints. Those commissioning evaluation therefore need to be well informed about the principles of evaluation and the implications for selecting particular research designs. They will also need to set criteria for assessing the capability of the various groups who submit tenders for an evaluation contract. Once appointed the evaluator/s will need to work closely with the commissioner/s, project team and other stakeholders. As with all partnership working, good communication, mutual respect and designation of roles and responsibilities are essential – an issue we will address in Chapter 5.

Clegg (2002) contends that little attention had been paid to 'the art of commissioning evaluation'. He notes the danger that those commissioning evaluation may over-extend the scope and have unrealistic expectations of what evaluators can achieve. He proposes that good commissioning is about 'creating a context in which evaluation can inform policy' and that the key issues are:

- modesty in expectation
- a focus away from accountability and attribution
- an orientation towards developing theory
- a concern to make a reality of multi-method approaches, so there is genuine triangulation and mutual illumination
- an openness to complexity and systems approaches.

The guidelines for commissioners of evaluation (UK Evaluation Society 2003b) also include having realistic expectations about what can be achieved and a clear specification of the purpose of and audience for any evaluation. Allan (2004) emphasizes the importance of being able to learn from the evaluation and notes the 'usefulness of an expectation for *constructive and critical appraisal* rather than an affirmation of good works'.

Summary: The big picture

Those commissioning evaluation and those responsible for carrying it out, along with any other stakeholders, will need to have a shared understanding about why the evaluation is needed and the questions it should address. A number of decision-making stages then follow which might be summarized as:

1 Purpose and scope
2 Design of the evaluation
3 Selection of indicators
4 Choice of data-gathering methods
5 Data analysis
6 Interpretation, presentation/publication and dissemination.

Many of the decisions at each stage are value-laden, and we will explore
alternative positions and their implications throughout the text. But for now,
we will conclude with Patton's (1997) key questions derived from Kipling's
Just So Stories (1902).

> I keep six honest serving-men
> (They taught me all I knew);
> Their names are What and Why and When
> And How and Where and Who.

Applied to evaluation, these questions become:

> Who is the evaluation for?
> What do we need to find out?
> Why do we want to find that out?
> When will the findings be needed?
> Where should we gather information?
> How will the results be used?

2 Evaluation – concepts and approaches

Overview

This chapter critically examines common approaches to evaluation. It includes:

- definition of evaluation and monitoring
- outcome evaluation, including experimental and quasi-experimental approaches
- achieving internal validity – triangulation and the judicial principle
- the importance of considering process and context
- realistic evaluation
- guiding principles.

What is evaluation?

There are a number of definitions of **evaluation** (see Box 2.1). A common feature of most definitions is assessing the effects of an intervention and whether goals have been achieved. However, this immediately raises the question of whether evaluation should focus on predetermined goals or be open to unanticipated outcomes. Further, a focus on predetermined goals presupposes that these have formally been identified at the planning stage of an intervention and that appropriate indicators of success have been developed. An additional issue to emerge from the definitions is the use of findings to assist in decision-making about future courses of action – either in relation to the development of specific programmes or by building the evidence base more generally. In contrast, **monitoring** has been defined as 'the systematic and continuous following, or keeping trace, of activities to ensure they are proceeding according to plan' (Feuerstein 1986: 184). The emphasis in monitoring is therefore on recording what has happened in terms of programme delivery, whereas evaluation is concerned with assessing what has been achieved and how any changes have come about.

Box 2.1 Definitions of evaluation

The systematic examination and assessment of the features of an initiative and its effects, in order to produce information that can be used by those who have an interest in its improvement or effectiveness. (WHO 1998: 3)

The critical assessment, on as objective a basis as possible, of the degree to which entire services or their component parts, fulfil stated goals. (St Leger et al. 1992: 1)

The purpose of evaluation is to 'measure the effects of a program against the goals it set out to accomplish as a means of contributing to the subsequent decision-making about the program and improving future program-making'. (Weiss 1972: 4; cited by Kaneko 1999: 433)

The aim of evaluation is to contribute towards solving practical problems, in terms of what works and why. It is about collecting information to inform action. Most of all it is about learning from experience. (Springett 2001a: 144)

Evaluation is essentially about determining the extent to which certain valued goals have been achieved. (Tones 1998: 52)

↻ Point for reflection

What various aspirations for evaluation are revealed by the differences in these definitions?

While acknowledging that evaluation research has much in common with other forms of research activity, Tones and Tilford (1994) draw on Smith (1975) to identify a number of points of distinction. These include the following:

- General research may serve a wide range of purposes, whereas the primary concern of evaluation is to assess the achievement of defined goals.
- Evaluation research is more likely to be commissioned by a client who may exert control over both the focus and the use of findings.
- Evaluation, especially if externally managed, may not be a major priority for participants.
- The greater emphasis on the use of evaluation findings to inform or influence decision-makers, in contrast to the general contribution to knowledge and understanding more typical of research.
- A wider diversity of stakeholders in evaluation and greater potential for conflict about the selection of appropriate indicators and the means of measuring their achievement.
- Potentially less control over the choice of evaluation research methods.
- Greater time constraints within evaluation research linked to the finite length of programmes.
- The findings of evaluation are principally to inform decision-makers, whereas research reports contribute to the development of more general academic knowledge and understanding.

Scott (1998) uses Herman *et al.*'s (1987) categorization to identify seven models of evaluation which are summarized in Table 2.1. While this usefully distinguishes between different types of evaluation and their respective primary focus, in practice it would be unusual to see these as discrete entities. A combination of the different models would be much more likely. However, recourse to such categorizations can be useful in raising awareness of the orientation of an evaluation and, indeed, unpicking the various purposes which different stakeholders may have for it.

Table 2.1 Models of evaluation

Evaluation model	Focus
Goal-orientated evaluation	Effectiveness, efficiency and economy of an intervention
Decision-orientated evaluation	Improve decision-making
Evaluation research	Providing explanations for outcomes
Responsive evaluation	Process of evaluation and perspectives of participants
Goal-free evaluation	Openness to achievements other than those prescribed by the intervention's aims and objectives
Alternative explanations	Alternatives to accepted descriptions about what is happening
Utilization-orientated evaluation	Utility of findings to different stakeholders

Notwithstanding any 'label' that might be attached, approaches clearly range from having a narrow focus on the achievement of pre-determined objectives through to understanding how change might have come about, the processes involved and openness to unanticipated effects. They also vary in the extent to which they are oriented towards meeting the needs of particular stakeholders.

There is an important point of distinction between summative and formative evolution. **Summative evaluation** is carried out towards the end of an intervention to assess achievements. While the emphasis tends to be on outcomes, it may also include a process element. Tones and Tilford (2001: 114) suggest that this is important for two reasons: firstly, to identify whether all the necessary components of an initiative have been put in place and provide a quality check to assist in interpreting levels of success or failure; secondly, to provide 'illuminative' insight into the processes involved. This type of 'illuminative evaluation' can offer explanations for achievements and identify key aspects of the design and delivery of interventions that would be of relevance to wider dissemination. It can complement answers to the question 'What did we achieve?' by providing information in response to 'How did we achieve it?', 'What did we learn?' and 'Would we do it the same way next time?'

While summative evaluation provides a retrospective analysis, **formative evaluation** is carried out at the same time as an initiative is being developed and implemented. It therefore has greater immediacy and relevance for those responsible for the delivery of interventions as it can provide essential information and feedback to guide developments. Formative evaluation is frequently concerned with processes. However, assessing the achievement of early outcomes will provide a check on progress towards targets and allow any necessary adjustment to the initiative to be made. Formative evaluation therefore has much in common with action research, defined by Cohen and Manion (1994: 192) as 'an on the spot procedure designed to deal with a concrete problem located in an immediate situation'.

Clearly users of evaluation evidence will require such evidence to be robust and expect to have a degree of confidence that claims of effectiveness and any reported change can actually be attributed to the intervention. There will be a number of major stakeholders in any evaluation (see Box 2.2).

Box 2.2 Stakeholders in evaluation

Funders
Manager
Project workers
Target population
Other practitioners working in a similar field
Policy-makers
Politicians
The wider public health community
Academics
Theoreticians

Point for reflection

How might the goals of funders differ from those of project workers and the target population?

It would be surprising among such a diverse group if there were not different views about the type of evidence which is held to be convincing and the nature of goals being assessed – especially if, as Tones suggests, evaluation addresses *valued* goals. Funders may be concerned with accountability and achieving value for money, project workers may be concerned with achieving health outcomes, whereas the target population may be concerned with whether their own perceived needs are being addressed. As Clegg (2002: 3) states: 'Commissioners know that different types of data will be well received by different stakeholders: the killer statistic for policy makers, the quotation for lobby groups and so on.' Chen (1990) suggests that evaluation should be:

- responsive to the needs of different stakeholders
- objective
- trustworthy
- generalizable.

Furthermore, there is the question of whether the emphasis should be on identifying *what* has been achieved or understanding *how* it has been achieved, that is, on assessing **outcomes** or the **process** of working towards them. We will consider process evaluation later in this chapter, but for now will focus on the achievement of outcomes.

Outcome evaluation

Outcome evaluation is concerned with documenting any change achieved as a result of an intervention. The terms **impact** and **outcome** are both used to refer to this change, and this can be the source of some confusion. Sentinella (2004: 8) defines outcomes as 'the changes that result from the programme'. The UK Evaluation Society (2003a) refers to impacts as 'A general term used to describe the effects of a programme on society. Impacts can be either positive or negative and foreseen or unforeseen.' However, 'impact' is generally used for more immediate effects (and the evaluation society reserves the term 'results' for initial effects) and 'outcome' for longer-term effects. Springett (1998a: 14) suggests that 'Impacts are the immediate outcomes and may not include an improvement in health. Outcomes are much longer term and more likely to be the product of the synergistic effect of many projects.' So these terms can be organized by time sequence and level of generality as follows:

results → impacts → outcomes

Despite general agreement on the above, some authors reverse the order and see outcomes leading to impacts (for example, Health Communication Unit 2006: 9). In the interest of simplicity, within this text we use the term 'outcome' and distinguish immediate, short- and longer-term outcomes. **Outputs**, in contrast, are the 'goods and services produced by the intervention' (UK Evaluation Society 2003a), that is, the range of activities and materials put in place to achieve the outcomes.

A fundamental issue is whether any reported change can actually be attributed to an intervention. How do the outcomes of the intervention compare with any **counterfactual** situation – the position that would have existed had the intervention not taken place? This question has been at the heart of debate about appropriate methods for evaluating health promotion interventions. The debate itself has been essentially epistemological (see Box 2.3), centring on the nature of the social world and ways of knowing reality. On the one hand there is the view, located in the positivist tradition, that it is possible to obtain an objective account of phenomena and establish causal relationships and pathways. This view supports the application of quantitative methods used within the natural sciences and experimental and quasi-experimental design. On the other hand, a constructivist or interpretivist position sees reality as constructed and acknowledges that there may be a range of different subjective meanings and interpretations. It typically draws on qualitative data-collection methods. We will outline the principles of experimental design before returning to the debate about evaluation methodology and considering the critiques of this approach.

Box 2.3 Definitions

Ontology is concerned with the nature of reality – what we believe to exist.

Epistemology is the theory of knowledge. It is essentially concerned with how we know what is true and the types of statement we accept to support this.

Methodology is the overall research strategy or approach. This derives from epistemological considerations, which would dictate the level of commitment to quantitative, qualitative or plural approaches and the selection of appropriate methods.

A paradigm is 'a worldview built on implicit assumptions, accepted definitions, comfortable habits, values defended as truths, and beliefs projected as reality. As such, paradigms are deeply embedded in the socialisation of adherents and practitioners: paradigms tell them what is important, legitimate and reasonable'. (Patton 1997: 267).

Experimental design

Experimental studies aim to establish causal relationships between phenomena. They explore the effect of one variable or set of variables (the so-called independent variable) on another (the dependent variable). In the case of evaluation research the independent variable is the intervention, and its effects constitute the dependent variable/s. A central concern is to ensure that any change can actually be attributed to the intervention and avoid so-called Type I error (see Box 2.5). In order to do this, experimental design attempts to exclude the effect of any factors other than the independent variable. It therefore minimizes confounding or 'muddling the picture so that it is difficult to discern what is causing what to happen' (Gomm *et al.* 2000: 45).

Box 2.4 A simple pre–post test

A school-based educational programme to improve awareness of the risks of unprotected sex delivered over a two-week period used a questionnaire to assess levels of awareness immediately before and after the programme.

Point for reflection

Could any reported change be attributed to the programme?

The example in Box 2.4 uses a simple pre–post test design to assess the effect of a programme. However, it could be that there is an extensive media campaign running at the same time and it would therefore be difficult to attribute any effects solely to the school-based intervention. Equally, the experience of completing the initial questionnaire may have raised awareness in itself or encouraged respondents to seek answers to queries that they were uncertain about. To avoid this type of problem experimental studies rely on the use of control groups based on the assumption that extraneous variables will affect intervention and control groups in the same way. Any reported differences between the two groups must therefore be due to the intervention.

Box 2.5 Types of error (from Basch and Gold 1986:300–1)

Common problems in drawing conclusions from evaluation research include:

Type I error	The wrong conclusion that an intervention has achieved significant change when it has actually failed to do so.
Type II error	The wrong conclusion that an intervention has failed to have a significant effect when it actually has done so.
Type III error	Judging that an intervention has failed when it was so poorly designed that it could not have achieved the desired effect.
Type IV error	Carrying out an evaluation of a programme that no-one cares about and is irrelevant to decision-making.
Type V error	The intervention is shown to have a statistically significant effect, but the change is so small as to have no practical significance.

Oakley (1998a) notes the early use of randomized controlled trials (RCTs) by educationalists in the USA, their later application in agriculture by researchers such as Fisher (1949) and their role in evaluating public policy interventions in the USA in the period 1960–1980. However it is in the field of medicine and drug trials that randomized trials have been most extensively used. An editorial in the *British Medical Journal* (Editor *BMJ* 1998) reported the 50th anniversary of the publication of the trial of streptomycin treatment for pulmonary tuberculosis – the first publication of a trial which fully reported the randomization process. The move to demonstrate effectiveness, spearheaded by influential thinkers such as Cochrane, has resulted in the widespread adoption of RCTs within medicine, although as we shall see later, this move has not been without its critics.

The randomized controlled double-blind trial

The 'gold standard' of experimental design has been held to be the randomized controlled double-blind trial. An outline of the process is provided in Figure 2.1. A representative sample is drawn from the wider study population and any appropriate inclusion and exclusion criteria applied. For example, in drug trials, patients with additional complicating conditions may be excluded. Informed consent is obtained from participants and they are then randomly allocated to intervention and control groups. Provided samples are sufficiently large, such random allocation should produce groups with similar characteristics – and the profiles of each group can be compared. If, however, it is deemed important to ensure equal representation within the two groups in relation to a particular characteristic such as gender or age, it is possible to stratify the sample into groups and then randomly allocate within each group.

Any appropriate baseline measures are carried out and then one group is exposed to the intervention while the control group either receives nothing or what was previously accepted as 'best practice'. Clearly any awareness of receiving an intervention (or not) will constitute a difference between the two groups over and above actual exposure to the intervention itself and may well have some effect. This so-called placebo effect in drug trials is well recognized. To compensate for this, subjects are usually not informed whether they are in the experimental or control arm of a trial and are essentially treated in the same way other than exposure to the substance under test. Ensuring that subjects are 'blind' to whether they are receiving the treatment being tested involves giving them a dummy drug or placebo in exactly the same form as the active drug and according to standardized protocols. The expectations of researchers and practitioners can also affect recorded outcomes. Gomm *et al.* (2000) cite research showing that even apparently physiological processes, such as the rate at which leg ulcers heal, can be influenced by practitioners' expectations. In double-blind trials, in addition to the subjects, practitioners and researchers are not made aware of whether participants are in the experimental or control arm until the end of the study.

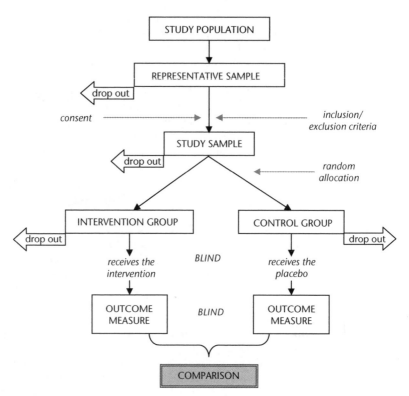

Figure 2.1 The randomized controlled double-blind trial

Comparison of any differences in outcome measures between the two groups will allow a judgement to be made about the effectiveness of the intervention. This assumes that there have been no major differences in **attrition** (i.e. people dropping out of the study) between the two groups – for example, people withdrawing from the experimental arm because of the experience of unpleasant side effects or because they are not experiencing any benefit.

The CONSORT statement (Moher *et al.* 2001) was developed to improve the quality of reports of RCTs. It recommends that the numbers of participants at each of the four main stages in an RCT are recorded – enrolment, intervention allocation, follow-up, analysis. This allows a so-called intention-to-treat analysis to be undertaken to avoid bias associated with non-random loss of participants. It deals with participants as though they were in the group to which they were originally allocated even if they refuse to comply with the treatment regimen.

Conventionally the comparison is made by a null hypothesis that the intervention has no effect and that there is no difference between intervention and control groups. The probability of obtaining the recorded results if the null hypothesis is true can be calculated using appropriate statistical tests. A low probability is indicative of a real difference between the groups and supports rejection of the null hypothesis and attribution of any difference to exposure to the intervention (see Box 2.6 for an example).

Box 2.6 *P*-values and the null hypothesis – an example

In a double-blind randomized trial of the effect of sunscreen use (Autier *et al.* 1999), 87 participants were randomly assigned to receive SPF10 or SPF30 sunscreen. They kept diaries of sun exposure and experience of skin reddening or sunburn. The mean cumulative sun exposures for the two groups were 58.2 hours and 72.6 hours, respectively ($P = 0.011$). The mean daily durations of sunbathing were 2.6 and 3.1 hours, respectively ($P = 0.0013$). The number of skin reddening or sunburn episodes was 159 in both groups ($P = 0.99$).

If the intervention had no effect, the probability of obtaining these differences in results for sun exposure is very low (around 1 in 100 for cumulative exposure and 1 in 1000 mean daily sunbathing duration). There must, therefore, be a real difference in behaviour between these groups which can be attributed to the use of the higher-factor sunscreen. The authors therefore concluded that 'use of higher SPF sunscreen seems to increase the duration of recreational sun exposure of young white Europeans'.

In contrast, the two groups are very similar with regard to skin reddening and episodes of sunburn. Based on the null hypothesis that there is no difference between these groups, the probability of getting the recorded incidences of episodes of sunburn is high. The null hypothesis is therefore upheld in this instance and it is very likely that there is no difference between the two groups. It can be concluded that the use of different levels of sun protection has no effect on incidence of sunburn.

Experimental methods scrutinized

The use of RCTs and experimental methods for evaluating the complex interventions more typical of public health has been questioned. Objections have been raised on epistemological and ideological grounds and also in relation to the practical applicability of this design. Even within the field of medicine, critics have noted that the use of RCTs should be restricted to situations which are simple and where there is uncertainty about outcomes (Charlton 1991; Black 1998). A summary of the deficiencies of drug trials was provided by a 1998 editorial in the *British Medical Journal* (see Box 2.7).

Box 2.7 Deficiencies of drug trials (Editor *BMJ* 1998)

Too small
Too short
Poor quality
Poorly presented
Methodological inadequacies
Few include adequate measures of quality of life
Cost data poorly presented
Ethical aspects often neglected
Views of participants are either not sought or forgotten
Participants often have limited understanding of what is happening
Poorly managed
Politics can hijack conclusions
Marketeers can use trials for their own ends

Control groups

In relation to the feasibility of using experimental design, it should be recognized that public health and health promotion interventions are fundamentally different from clinical interventions. As we noted in Chapter 1, they frequently involve complex multi-sectoral and multi-level approaches and tend to be targeted at populations, communities or groups rather than individuals. A defining feature of RCTs and experimental design is the random allocation of individuals to experimental and control groups. However, efforts to improve health – and particularly those that are known to be most effective – do not take the neatly packaged form which would allow random allocation of individuals to intervention and control groups. As Nutbeam (1998: 36) notes, 'the artificial assignment of individuals in communities to intervention and control groups is not only often impractical, but frequently impossible as it places quite unrealistic constraints on the evaluation design'. Bonnell's case study provides an extreme example of the lengths some researchers will go to in their attempts to use experimental designs. He reports a study into the effectiveness of group counselling for HIV prevention for gay men which went as far as changing the form of the intervention in order to avoid problems with recruitment and retention during the trial. One of those involved commented: 'We did have to tailor the intervention to some extent. And that isn't really what I think should happen with sexual health; we should be finding research, means of research, that fit with the intervention' (Bonnell 2002: 326). The change involved reducing the length of the intervention and flying in the face of earlier evidence that several sessions were needed – a clear case of the evaluation 'tail' wagging the intervention 'dog' in programme planning!

Instead of randomly assigning individuals, it may be more feasible to allocate naturally occurring units such as schools, hospitals or communities. These are usually referred to as quasi-experimental studies in order to distinguish them from true experimental studies in which the individual is the unit of assignment. The term 'comparison group' is also used instead of control group – although not universally so. Many of the large-scale community intervention trials have involved random allocation of matched communities to intervention and comparison groups – for example, COMMIT (see Box 2.8). However, this raises the question of what the 'unit' of study is. Clearly if a whole community is regarded as one intervention unit – the equivalent of one individual taking a drug in a drug trial – then the scale of community intervention trials becomes enormous if sufficient numbers are to be included for comparative purposes. This is clearly beyond the capacity of most projects and is comparatively rare within evaluation practice. Such trials take on the form of 'demonstration projects', for example the major heart health demonstration projects such as North Karelia, Stamford Three-Community and Five-City, Minnesota and Pawtucket (Shea and Basch 1990). Nutbeam (1998) is critical of approaches in which the 'unit of intervention' and 'assignment' is a whole group or population and the unit of observation remains the individual.

Box 2.8 The Community Intervention Trial for Smoking Cessation (COMMIT) – a quasi-experimental study

Eleven matched pairs of communities were selected to reflect the range of communities across North America. The pairs were geographically separate to avoid contamination and each of the pair was randomly assigned to intervention or comparison group. The programme aimed to establish a social climate that was not supportive of tobacco use. It included 58 specified activities which were delivered by local staff and volunteers through four main channels in the intervention arm of the study:

- media and community events
- health care providers
- workplaces and other organizations
- smoking cessation resources.

The effect of the programme was assessed by comparing rates of quitting among different types of smoker (heavy, light to moderate) between the two study groups (COMMIT Research Group 1991).

Points for reflection

What do you see as the major strengths of this study?

What are the potential weaknesses?

What epistemological position is reflected in your assessment?

Approaches which do not involve randomization can also be used and take the form of 'natural experiments'. However, groups which elect to adopt interventions may differ in a number of ways from those which do not. This raises the issue of comparability of the groups and poses a threat to internal validity. Furthermore, in situations where the community itself has recognized the need for change and the motive force comes from the community, it is virtually impossible to find an adequate control group. Green and Tones (1999) have argued that where such community commitment is an important contributory factor we should acknowledge and attempt to understand its contribution rather than control for its presence.

Contamination can also be a problem, especially with large-scale interventions and those that take place over long periods of time. Unless populations are widely spaced geographically it is difficult to maintain impermeable boundaries between intervention and control groups. Moreover, control or reference groups will not remain frozen in time and developments may well take place within them which may compromise their use as controls. For example, Nutbeam et al. (1993) noted that the reference groups used in evaluating the Heartbeat Wales programme independently set up their own heart health initiatives.

Detecting change

A major challenge for evaluators is picking out any change attributable to the intervention from the background 'noise' of other changes and trends. Type II error is said to occur when we fail to detect such change (see Box 2.5). It can arise because the type of measurement used is insufficiently sensitive to detect change or because we are trying to measure the wrong thing. We will consider appropriate outcome indicators more fully in Chapter 3. However, it is worth noting here that experimental and quasi-experimental designs in public health frequently rely on epidemiological indicators such as changes in morbidity and mortality. This need not be the case, but the association reflects a common epistemology underpinning the selection of methods and outcome measures. Given the plethora of factors which will affect morbidity and mortality, any change due to a particular intervention is likely to be small, difficult to detect and, indeed, may not appear for many years. This can be particularly problematic for small-scale studies which may not have sufficient power to reveal a significant difference between intervention and control groups even when they achieve what practitioners might agree is a meaningful level of change. Green and Tones (1999) caution that with infinitely large samples it is possible to establish significant differences when the actual change is too small to have any practical relevance (Type V error). This confuses practical significance with statistical significance (Basch and Gold 1986). Practitioners should therefore be involved in establishing what level of change could reasonably be anticipated.

Nutbeam (1998) refers to the fact that major community intervention trials such as the cardiovascular programmes and COMMIT smoking cessation trials have been disappointing in terms of the recorded net impact on targeted risk factors. Positive results have been recorded in both intervention and comparison groups and programmes seem to have had little effect over and above these positive secular trends. One explanation he offers is that the positive trends in smoking, physical activity and nutrition have been achieved as the result of 'sustained public health activism over the last three decades' (Nutbeam 1998: 37). The effects of relatively short-term localized interventions can therefore be overshadowed by such sustained activity.

The quality and nature of the intervention

Much of the debate about the evaluation of interventions to promote health focuses on evaluation methodology and tends to overlook the quality of the intervention. Speller *et al.* (1997) contend that inclusion of studies in systematic reviews of evidence is based on the quality of research and not the quality of the intervention. Returning to the notion of error (see Box 2.5), Type III error is said to occur when a programme or approach is judged to be ineffective, but the programme itself was inadequate either in its design or delivery. Well-designed health promotion programmes should be based on relevant theory and other empirical evidence. Programmes should be adequately resourced and of a sufficient level of intensity to achieve change. They should also be fully and faithfully implemented. Wulf (1993), for example, noted the 34 per cent of schools providing the Drug Abuse Resistance Education programme did not include all the lessons and 42 per cent had made modifications to the programme. Such monitoring information about the fidelity of programme implementation is clearly essential for interpreting findings.

There is an important point of distinction between effectiveness and efficacy. **Effectiveness** is used to refer to achievements under normal conditions, whereas Brook and Lohr (1985) use the term **efficacy** to refer to effectiveness under ideal conditions. Somewhat paradoxically, concern to avoid Type III error by ensuring that programmes are delivered in their 'ideal' form limits the generalizability of findings to more naturalistic settings in which programme fidelity is likely to be much lower. As we will see below, to avoid compromising external validity (see Box 2.9) some understanding of process is needed.

Box 2.9 Validity

This is the extent to which an evaluation actually measures what it sets out to measure. Internal validity is essentially concerned with detecting change and being able to attribute it to the intervention. External validity concerns the extent to which evaluation findings are applicable to other situations and contexts.

↻ **Points for reflection**

What factors might compromise

- internal validity?
- external validity?

Bonnell (2002) makes the point that new clinical interventions are subjected to preliminary testing in relation to their effects – both beneficial and unwanted side effects – before they can be accepted for formal trial. This rarely happens in relation to social interventions, and yet if we are to avoid Type III error there should be some assessment of whether proposed interventions are acceptable, sufficiently comprehensive and meet identified needs.

Ideological and epistemological considerations

The core values of health promotion are participation, empowerment and collaboration (Tilford *et al.* 2003). Experimental approaches which objectify individuals are inconsistent with these core values. A key feature of many health promotion interventions is the active involvement of individuals and communities. The logical extension of this approach to intervention is that it should equally be applied to evaluation. Appropriate evaluation should therefore include 'the notions of participation, community control and respect for people, not as unthinking objects of research, but as partners in knowledge development' (Springett 2001a: 139). Furthermore, interpretivists would reject the positivist position that it is possible to reach a single objective truth and would subscribe to the view that individuals meaningfully construct reality. Alternative positions are therefore possible, and experimental evaluations which focus on pre-determined outcomes would overlook these. Qualitative insights are held to be important not only in identifying the range of possible outcomes, but also in understanding the process of programme delivery and change.

The intensity of the debate about positivist and constructivist approaches to evaluation has been such that the term 'paradigm wars' has been used to refer to it (Pawson and Tilley 1997; Tones and Green 2004). However, other evaluators take a more pragmatic position and use a combination of methods derived from both camps. The key issue is whether such pragmatism is a knee-jerk reaction to the possibly ill-conceived demands of stakeholders or a considered response to the evaluation problem. Patton (1997: 296), in developing the case for utilization-focused evaluation, argues as follows:

> I disagree, then, that philosophical assumptions necessarily require allegiance by evaluators to one paradigm or the other. Pragmatism can overcome seemingly logical contradictions . . . the flexible and open evaluator

can view the same data from the perspective of each paradigm and can help adherents of either paradigm interpret data in more than one way.

Public health is committed to the value of health and achieving change to improve health and tackle inequalities. Clearly there will be some variation in how health is defined, ranging from a narrow focus on prevention of disease to a more holistic view encompassing positive well-being. Professional groups such as Health Promotion, as we have noted, are committed to particular ways of working – for example, ways which are participatory and empowering. A further issue is whether the source of the problem is held to reside with individuals and their health behaviour or the wider social determinants of health and ill-health. Springett (2001a: 142) draws on the work of Habermas and Heidegger to identify the relevance to health promotion and public health of placing emphasis on 'the relationship between organism and the environment, on context, on the whole being greater than the sum of the parts; on connexions and synergy; on emergent systems, complexity and non-linear causality'. Evaluating public health interventions cannot, therefore, be value-free. Research in the critical realist tradition does not aim to be neutral, but is committed to challenging oppressive social structures. It draws on interpretivist approaches, but at the same time accepts the actual existence of structures and processes which shape individual experience (Connelly 2001).

Public health interventions are complex and do not conform to a simple input–output model. To address this, evaluation needs to draw on both qualitative and quantitative methods. It requires a methodologically plural approach which combines methods traditionally associated with different epistemological positions. Notwithstanding widespread support for and adoption of this approach, there remain critics. For some, alternative epistemological positions reflect real differences in views about the nature of reality. For example Guba and Lincoln (1989: 17) argue that 'no accommodation is possible between positivist and constructivist belief systems'. In contrast, while acknowledging the contribution of constructivist interpretations, Pawson and Tilley (1997: 23), arguing from a realist perspective, recognize that there are structures and institutional features which are 'independent of the individual's reasoning and desires' which would therefore be open to other forms of inquiry. Other objections have related more to practice. Milburn *et al.* (1995), for example, note that the combination of methods is often pragmatic and unreflective, and insufficient attention is given to the actual way in which findings are combined.

Achieving internal validity: triangulation and the judicial principle

Notwithstanding the association between randomized trials and scientific rigour, we have argued that such experimental and quasi-experimental methods have little, if any, role in evaluating public health and health promotion interventions in view of their serious limitations in relation to their:

- practical feasibility
- tendency to focus on individual behaviour rather than macro-level determinants of health
- ability to deal with complex interventions
- ability to address the complexity of change
- utility in informing policy and practice.

Barreto (2005: 346) argues that if public health were required to conform with the same principles as those used for evaluating biomedical interventions (the RCT), it would no longer be feasible 'for public health to propose interventions in areas such as the environment, education, behaviour, and principally social interventions such as those concerning health inequalities'. An example of the way undue reliance on this type of evidence can influence recommendations for practice and lead to individually orientated solutions rather than addressing the more fundamental social causes of problems is provided by Davey Smith *et al.* (2005). They quote the evaluation group set up for the Independent Inquiry into Inequalities in Health: 'Our recommendations are quite medical because those are the sort that tend to have evidence behind them' (Laurance 1998). We risk being trapped in a false circular logic which dictates that sound evidence conforms with experimental principles, such principles can only be applied to simple interventions, acceptable evidence only accumulates on simple interventions, so we can only recommend simple interventions.

We therefore concur with WHO that the complexity of public health and health promotion interventions makes methods used for more simple clinical interventions unsuitable and 'The use of randomised controlled trials to evaluate health promotion initiatives is, in most cases, inappropriate, misleading and unnecessarily expensive' (WHO 1998: 5).

How then are we to avoid Type I error and ensure internal validity? How can we avoid the problems of positivist approaches and yet still produce evaluation findings that are rigorous and usefully contribute to the evidence base?

Triangulation can be used to enhance validity by drawing on different perspectives to corroborate findings. The term has its origins in surveying which accurately establishes a location by taking bearings from two or more positions. Triangulation can take a number of different forms (Denzin 1970):

- data triangulation makes use of different types of data
- investigator triangulation involves a number of different researchers
- theory triangulation draws on different theories/models
- methodological triangulation combines different methodological positions and makes use of different methods.

It is perhaps worth noting, however, that triangulation conforms with 'a positivist frame of reference which assumes a single (undefined) reality' (Silverman 1985: 105). This remains problematic for interpretive researchers whose primary concern is with meaning or, to be more precise, the range of different meanings and interpretations (Tones and Tilford 2001).

Notwithstanding such concerns, faith in the validity of findings will be increased if consistent observations emerge from different sources.

Given the nature of social interventions, establishing absolute proof of their effectiveness remains elusive. Yet sound evaluation evidence is needed to inform decisions. In day-to-day life major decisions are often taken in the absence of certainty by weighing up information. Even in the clinical situation Black (1998: 25) has suggested that 'we are more commonly persuaded by a balance of likelihoods than we are driven forward by the iron laws of evidence'. Tesh proposes that

> We just have to hold facts lightly, continually testing them against experience and logic, recognising their connection to the rules and context within which they appear, and most importantly, never ceasing to scrutinise the values which necessarily permeate them. (Tesh 1988: 177; cited by Baum 1995: 462)

The 'judicial principle' has been proposed as a way of applying this thinking to weighing up evaluation evidence (Tones 1997; Green and Tones 1999; Tones and Green 2004).

Essentially the judicial principle relies on triangulation. It suggests that decisions taken about evaluation evidence could be taken in the same way as in courts of law. Evidence from different sources is presented and decisions about guilt or innocence are based on this. Evaluation evidence could be assessed similarly. Further, different levels of certainty could be employed – **beyond reasonable doubt** in situations when a high level of certainty is needed, and **on the balance of probabilities** when there are less stringent demands.

Process and context: the quest for illumination

We note in our earlier definition of evaluation that its principal function is to inform decision-making. Bonnell (2002: 322) looks at the utility of RCTs and how useful the findings are in 'informing decisions made about how services are planned and implemented'. One of the major criticisms of experimental approaches to evaluation is that concern to achieve internal validity may compromise external validity, that is the extent to which the findings might apply to other communities and populations. Further, there is also a well-known tendency for people who are aware they are being researched to behave differently – the so-called Hawthorne effect.

Kaneko's (1999) review of the COMMIT trial referred to in Box 2.8 noted that although the aggregate data for the whole study showed no significant effect on heavy smokers and a small, although significant, effect on light to moderate smokers, detailed examination of the matched pairs showed considerable variation (see Table 2.2). In some there were significant positive effects, whereas in others the comparison group appeared to do better than the experimental group. Rather than attempting to explore alternative explanations of why these differences occurred, the evaluators focused solely on the intervention as the causal influence.

Table 2.2 Numbers of heavy smokers and fraction quitting in COMMIT intervention and comparison communities

Pair	Intervention community		Comparison community		Percentage difference
	Number	% quitting	Number	% quitting	
1	442	13.9	435	20.5	−6.6
2	531	16.3	489	20.2	−3.9
3	475	16.4	464	16.3	0.2
4	428	20.4	497	24.9	−4.5
5	440	18.3	458	16.0	2.2
6	450	16.4	454	18.6	−2.2
7	432	26.2	451	23.0	3.2
8	455	19.3	434	16.9	2.4
9	455	21.5	462	12.7	8.8
10	426	13.6	451	17.2	−3.6
11	442	15.5	448	18.9	−3.4
Total	4976	18.0	5043	18.7	−0.7

Source: Derived from COMMIT Research Group (1995), cited by Kaneko (1999).

In principle, a number of differences may exist which would influence the achievement of outcomes:

• fidelity in the delivery of programmes
• demographic factors which impact on health-related behaviour
• perceived relevance and acceptability of programmes to different communities
• differences in the way the communities perceive and receive the intervention
• the existence of other conditions supportive of change.

⟳ Point for reflection

What additional information would have been relevant to interpreting the findings of the study?

Pawson and Tilley (1997) are critical of the **successionist** logic underpinning experimental and quasi-experimental approaches. This assumes that cause is external and will consistently produce the same effect. Alternatively, **generative** theory of causation holds that there are causal relationships that may be linked to an external event, but that also depend on internal features or characteristics. It therefore tries to understand why programmes work. In the COMMIT example, why did the intervention work with some communities and not others? The learning derived from exploring these differences would more usefully inform the wider application of the programme and also our understanding of how change occurs. Sanderson (2000) draws on complexity theory to suggest that the relationship between inputs and outputs will not be linear, but will be context-dependent. Different aspects of the policy environment, as well as different programmes, will interact. A number of elements may need to be in place before a programme can be effective. Change will therefore not be incremental. An intervention may have no effect at all until all the other necessary conditions are in place and, once they are, may produce very rapid change.

We need to know not only if a programme is effective, but also with what type of population, in what context and how it works. We need to look inside the **black box** (Pawson and Tilley 1997; Tones and Tilford 2001) between inputs and outcomes to explore what is taking place. Rather than strip away any contextual factors as potential sources of confounding, we need to understand how they influence programme delivery and success. Outcome evaluation, therefore, cannot be separated from process evaluation. The analogy has been used that focusing solely on outcomes is rather like a theatre critic judging a performance on the basis of the applause without having seen it (Parlett and Hamilton 1972). Futhermore, Pawson and Myhill (2001) note the complex interaction between process and outcomes – see Box 2.10.

Box 2.10 Pawson and Myhill's Evaluation Lesson 3

Programme outcomes are the result of programme processes and evaluations are always enhanced to the extent that the study of one supports the understanding of the other. Programmes dependent on elaborate social processes will always generate a complex footprint of outcome. Anticipating and understanding these patterns demands a partnership of 'process' and 'outcome' evaluation, and requires the use of both quantitative and qualitative methods. (Pawson and Myhill 2001, cited in Sentinella 2004: 68)

The aims of process evaluation in published work have been summarized by Nutbeam (1998) as follows:

- Programme reach: did the programme reach all the target population?
- Programme integrity: was the programme implemented as planned?
- Programme acceptability: is the programme acceptable to the target population?

While such information on the quality and implementation of the programme is essential to interpreting findings, it does not go far enough in terms of fully understanding the process of change. In addition to commenting on the intervention itself, process evaluation should also focus on how the intervention is received and achieves (or fails to achieve) change.

A realist approach

Pawson and Tilley (1997) have been influential in developing realist approaches to evaluation. At the heart of their approach is the view that outcomes are the product of complex mechanisms which may be triggered by an intervention. Outcomes are also heavily influenced by contextual factors. This might be summarized as follows:

context + mechanisms → outcomes

The key features of realistic evaluation are:

1 It subscribes to a generative theory of causation. Change is not produced externally, but interventions release the potential for change and it is this process that needs to be understood.
2 It requires ontological depth. Evaluation should penetrate further than simple input–output relationships to understand how change occurs.
3 Evaluators need to consider causal mechanisms.
4 The context within which causal mechanisms operate should be understood.
5 Outcomes are important, not simply to confirm success or failure, but in terms of the multiple outcomes that can arise from the context–mechanism configuration.
6 The context–mechanism–outcome configuration provides information about what works for whom and under what circumstances. The learning derived from such an approach is therefore transferable.
7 Evaluators should work through an interchanging 'teacher–learner' relationship with key stakeholders rather than treat them as respondents.
8 Evaluation occurs within open systems. Interventions take place in a changing social world and their effectiveness may be influenced by changing contexts.

Summary: Guiding principles

Having considered a range of approaches to and perspectives about evaluation, what is our own position? We would endorse WHO's (1998: 3) commitment to using multiple methods and 'employing a broad a range of information gathering processes'. This view is not born of pragmatism but reflects our recognition of the value of methodological pluralism. It accepts that positivist and interpretivist approaches can and should be combined and offer complementary insights. It also accepts that establishing absolute proof is, in the case of most public health interventions, unrealistic and that, in line with the 'judicial principle', sound decisions can be based on the 'balance of probabilities'. We are also heavily influenced by the scientific realist approach developed by Pawson and Tilley (1997) which emphasizes the importance of understanding the way in which mechanisms and context contribute to outcomes.

Our key principles for evaluating public health interventions are set out below:

1 *Purpose*. Evaluation should be carried out for a purpose. That purpose should be agreed by the key stakeholders, made explicit at the outset and in reporting any findings.

2 *Practicality*. Evaluation should be of practical relevance both to those involved in delivering the programme and the wider public health community. The understanding generated should enhance the capacity to improve the health of individuals and communities.

3 *Process*. Knowing how change comes about and under what circumstances change is achieved is as important as identifying outcomes. Evaluation should therefore consider process as well as outcomes.

4 *Peripheral (contextual) factors*. Evaluation should consider the influence of contextual factors on ways of working and the achievement of outcomes.

5 *Probing*. Evaluation should attempt to provide more than simple input–output findings and probe beneath the surface to offer explanations of more general relevance and contribute to the development of theory.

6 *Plurality*. Evaluation should use multiple methods for gathering information.

7 *Participation*. Evaluation should draw on a range of perspectives to define its scope and methods and seek to involve all those with a legitimate interest.

8 *Plausibility*. The findings should make sense to major stakeholder groups and be consistent with their experience.

9 *Power*. Evaluation necessarily takes place within existing power structures. Evaluation should recognize but not be constrained by these. It should seek to include the lay perspective and operate in ways which are empowering.

10 *Politics*. Evaluation is essentially political. The findings will inform decisions at a number of different levels (project, organization, local policy, national policy) and contribute to the evidence base more generally.

3 Evidence and indicators of success

Overview

This chapter looks at the development and use of indicators to measure success and includes:

- the definition of success
- the importance of objectives
- types of indicator – outcome, intermediate and process
- the Theory of Change approach
- logic models
- gathering information.

Introduction

Notwithstanding the broader purposes of evaluation discussed in Chapter 2, evaluation is essentially concerned with assessing whether or not interventions have been successful. Speller *et al.* (1997: 363) emphasize the need to include 'the impact of interventions on systems and organisational developments as well as change in individual behaviour'. We have already considered the question of whether any gains can be attributed to an intervention and now turn our attention to two further key questions:

- How do we define success?
- How can we measure or assess success?

Furthermore if, as we have argued, understanding the process is also essential, we need to be able to identify key elements of the process.

This chapter begins by considering parameters for judging success and the centrality of clear goals and indicators. While identifying overarching goals is relatively straightforward, it is our experience that many projects struggle to specify how they will know when they have achieved them or reached the various stages in the change pathway leading towards them. Identifying appropriate outcome and process indicators is fundamental to evaluation together with understanding the ways in which interventions lead to change. The use of Theory of Change and logic models is considered as a means of approaching this task. The chapter concludes with a brief discussion of data collection.

Defining success

As we noted in Chapter 2, the term **effectiveness** is generally used to refer to the extent to which interventions have achieved their goals. In contrast, **efficacy** is concerned with effectiveness under ideal conditions (Brook and Lohr 1985). It assumes that interventions are delivered under optimal conditions and implemented with complete fidelity. Tones and Green (2004) refer to the 'efficacy paradox' which alerts us to the fact that it is unlikely that the levels of success achieved by such 'ideal' interventions will be replicated when programmes are implemented under more 'normal' working conditions.

The concept of **efficiency** incorporates the notion of **relative** effectiveness, that is, how effective a particular intervention is compared with others. While by no means necessarily the case, such comparisons frequently include consideration of costs, to which we will return below.

It cannot be assumed that all the outcomes of a programme are directly attributable to its effects. The distinction between **outcomes** and **effects** is well summarized by Granger (1998). An outcome is 'a measure of the variables that follow all or some of the intervention', whereas an effect is 'the outcome minus an estimate of what would have occurred without the intervention'. Some understanding of the 'counterfactual situation' – the position if the intervention had not taken place – is needed to provide a good estimate of effects.

Time-scale

Reference to time-scale is needed in planning evaluations, defining objectives and interpreting any reported outcomes. What can reasonably be expected to be achieved within the allotted time? The full benefits of health promotion interventions, framed either as positive well-being or as disease prevention, may take many years to develop (Parry-Langdon *et al.* 2003). For example, it could take decades for the full effect of a physical activity programme for young women to emerge in relation to the incidence of coronary heart disease. Clearly this is beyond the scope of most evaluations, which therefore have to rely on appropriate intermediate and short-term indicators – an issue to which we will return later. There may also be a time-lag between intervention and the emergence of behavioural effects. For example, a cancer education programme at school may increase the uptake of breast screening in adult life. Furthermore, some programmes – independently of any effects they may have in their own right – may enhance the response to a subsequent programme. The school cancer education programme could later enhance the response to a breast screening programme targeted at adults.

Green (1977) refers to the **delay** of impact noted above as the **sleeper effect**. The phenomenon of **decay** in impact once a programme has come to an end is well recognized. For example, an evaluation of the early SMARTRISK

Table 3.1 Behavioural intention following an injury prevention programme

Behavioural intention	% reporting always or often		
	Before	After	6 weeks
Wear a cycle helmet	27.0	45.6	29.4
Wear a seat belt (front passenger)	85.6	91.0	84.4
Wear a seat belt (back passenger)	69.8	80.2	74.4
Cross in a safe place	55.6	68.7	60.4
Wait for the light	45.4	60.1	49.7

Source: Green and Camidge (2001).

Heroes injury prevention programme for young people in the UK found an initial positive improvement in behavioural intention followed by some decline at the 6-week follow-up, as shown in Table 3.1. Green refers to this decay in impact over time as the **backsliding effect**. He also identifies three additional time-dependent effects:

• Borrowing from the future or **trigger effect**. The effect of a programme may be overestimated if it initiates change that would have happened anyway. The intervention merely brings forward or hastens change. Referring to the example in Box 3.1, if those attending for screening are those who would have attended in the reasonably near future anyway, the initial gains may be offset by a reduction in attendance at a later point, leading to a reduced or even zero net effect.

• Adjusting for secular trends or **historical effect**. Gains may be apparent following an intervention, but what proportion can actually be attributed to the intervention itself? General changes in behaviour patterns, either positive or negative, will need to be accounted for so that gains are not overestimated or, equally, underestimated. The use of control or reference groups, referred to in Chapter 2, can be useful for this purpose. However, it presupposes that change is taking place at the same rate in both groups.

• Backlash from cessation of programme or **contrast effect**. The termination of a programme, especially if this is premature or if the way the programme was implemented has alienated the community in any way, may result in a backlash. Initial gains may be followed by a reversal, resulting in a worse position than at the beginning of the programme.

Box 3.1 Chlamydia screening

A mass media programme to promote chlamydia screening among young women was followed by an immediate increase in attendance.

↻ Points for reflection

Has the programme been effective? What additional information would you like to have access to?

How much can be achieved?

One of the major difficulties in setting targets is knowing what level of change can reasonably be expected and identifying what criteria of success could be set. A **criterion** is 'a standard by which something may be judged or evaluated' (Feuerstein 1986: 183). It establishes a threshold for determining success. If there are well-documented time trends, these can be extrapolated and a target can be set greater than that which would have occurred anyway.

However, this type of information is frequently not available. Many evaluations therefore have to rely on loose estimates (and even guestimates) or, as is frequently the case, overlook the issue by simply reporting changes without reference to criteria. In some extreme instances, there is even uncertainty about which direction of change should be associated with success – see the example in Box 3.2.

Box 3.2 Utilization of services

One of the objectives of a Healthy Living Centre focusing on mental health was to achieve appropriate usage of general practitioner services.

Points for reflection

Would an increase or decrease in consultations be expected if the Centre were successful?

How useful is service utilization data in assessing the effectiveness of the Centre?

Furthermore, change within communities is rarely linear. Green and Richard (1993) suggest that secular trends in health behaviours follow the classic S-shaped curve of communication of innovations theory (Figure 3.1). The steepness of the curve is indicative of the rate of adoption and the shape is due to the differential rate of adoption among the groups that make up a population. Programmes which are implemented at an early stage in the general diffusion of secular trends are more likely to be able to demonstrate significant change than those which are at a later stage. The final group of 'laggards' is particularly resistant to change and achieving success with such groups is challenging. Green and Richard locate the start points of the major heart health demonstration projects in relation to the innovation–diffusion curve. The North Karelia Project in Finland was at the very beginning, whereas the Stanford Three-Community Study, Stanford Five-City Project and Minnesota Heart Health Projects, all in the USA, were at successively later stages and demonstrated correspondingly less impressive outcomes.

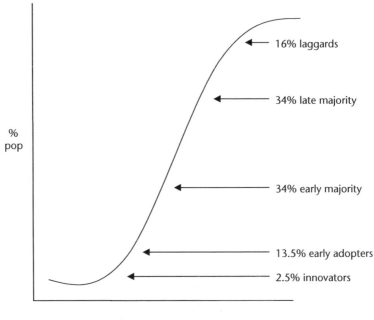

Figure 3.1 The S-shaped diffusion curve (Rogers and Shoemaker 1971)

Notwithstanding differential behaviour among adopter groups, a ceiling effect will also exist in a purely mathematical sense. In populations with a large proportion already demonstrating a particular positive health behaviour there is less capacity to demonstrate any improvement. To compensate for this, Green and Lewis proposed an effectiveness index (EI) based on the formula

$$EI = \frac{P_2 - P_1}{100 - P_1}$$

where P_1 represents the percentage reporting adoption before an intervention, and P_2 the percentage reporting adoption after the intervention.

A further consideration in predicting what might be a reasonable magnitude of change is the number of stages to be successfully negotiated prior to the achievement of the desired outcome. Tones and Tilford (2001) provide an example using the mass media 'Slip, Slap, Slop' campaign to reduce skin cancer. The message of the campaign was 'slip' on a T-shirt, 'slap' on a hat, 'slop' on the sun cream. The sequence required, known as the 'hierarchy of communication effects', is outlined in Table 3.2. If we reasonably assume that at each stage only a proportion will go on to the next stage then anticipated levels of success will decline with each succeeding stage. For example, if only 30 per cent are aware of the message and 85 per cent of this group understand the message then only 25.5 per cent of the total population will understand the message.

Table 3.2 Hierarchy of communication effects

Stage	Effect	Cumulative totals
1. Aware of the message	30%	30%
2. Understand the message	85%	25.5%
3. Believe the message and have a positive attitude	31%	7.9%
4. Acquire relevant skill	40%	3.16%
5. Adopt the behaviour	50%	1.58%

Source: adapted from Tones and Tilford (2001: 129).

McGuire (1981), cited by Tones and Tilford (2001), refers to the 'attenuated effects fallacy' when the evaluator fails to take account of links in the input–output chain and the fact that the probability of achieving each stage is a product of the probabilities of reaching the previous stages. The final level of adoption of 1.58 per cent in the hypothetical example provides a salutary warning for evaluators and programme planners against over-ambitious expectations of change. Furthermore, the magnitude of any change is likely to be greater the earlier or more proximal position it occupies in the sequence of change. It follows, then, that demonstrating change is relatively easier for the earlier stages in a causally linked sequence.

Economic considerations

Economic evaluations involve identifying and giving a monetary cost to inputs and outcomes. Accounting for all costs is clearly a highly complex undertaking. Godfrey (2001) notes that a narrow perspective on costs would include only the immediate, direct costs of an intervention and its benefits. However, unless all costs and consequences are included a distorted view of value for money can easily emerge. Identifying these comprehensively and with any degree of certainty is challenging. This is particularly so for interventions typical of public health, which may draw on resources from a number of different sectors and the community itself and achieve a broader range of health and social benefits than simply disease prevention outcomes.

A further challenge is how to compare interventions which may yield widely dissimilar outcomes – for example, smoking cessation programmes and breast screening. The quality-adjusted life year (QALY) is frequently used and combines length and quality of life into one index. It assumes that if good-quality life is given a value of 1 then poor-quality life is worth less than 1. Assessing quality of life in this context is based essentially on negative health states such as the presence of diseases, disability or poor functioning (for more detail, see Bowling 1997a, 1997b; Edgar *et al.* 1998; Euroqol n.d.), and there is considerable debate about how to measure quality of life objectively.

QALYs have further been challenged because they can result in prioritization based on capacity to benefit rather than on actual need. They systematically favour interventions targeted at the young who clearly have most to gain in terms of additional years, and are hence fundamentally ageist.

Economic evaluation is a specialist field and a full discussion is beyond the scope of this volume. A range of further guidance is available (for example, Tolley 1993; Miller 2001; Meadows n.d.; Byford *et al.* 2003). However, it is worth summarizing the different types of full economic evaluation identified by Godfrey (2001) and briefly considering some of the arguments about the relevance of economic evaluation to public health.

- *Cost minimization analysis.* This compares the costs of alternative interventions assuming that the outcomes of each – both direct and indirect – will be the same. On the basis of this comparison, the lower-cost option can be identified.
- *Cost-effectiveness analysis.* The costs of the programme are quantified in monetary terms and the benefits are identified, ideally as some quantifiable unit such as reduced incidence of a disease or number of life years saved, although no monetary value is assigned to these. It allows the costs to be calculated per unit of achievement – see Box 3.3. For example, within the field of smoking cessation, the cost of providing nicotine replacement therapy per person giving up smoking for 1 year or more could be compared with the cost of general practitioners providing advice to stop smoking during normal consultations per person giving up smoking for 1 year or more.

Box 3.3 Statins and smoking cessation compared

The Wanless Report (Wanless 2002) looked critically at the costs and effectiveness of different public health interventions. The NHS expenditure on statins (drugs that reduce cholesterol) is in the region of £500 million per year. The cost-effectiveness of smoking cessation is between £212 and £873 per QALY, in contrast to between £4000 and £8000 per QALY for statins.

↻ Points for reflection

Should the NHS continue to put this level of resources into statins?

Can this type of information alone guide decisions?

- *Cost–utility analysis.* This incorporates some consideration of the value or utility of the outcomes. For example, rather than just identifying years of life gained, the use of QALYs allows some adjustment to be made to reflect quality of life.
- *Cost–benefit analysis.* Costs are assigned to both the provision of the intervention and all the benefits that accrue from it. This means that 'the

benefits must be translated into a [monetary] value' (Health Communication Unit 2006: 9). The two can then be compared, often as a cost–benefit ratio. For example, a study by Wang and Macera (2005) compared the cost of bike/pedestrian trails, including construction, maintenance and the equipment needed for using the trails, with the benefits of reduced health care costs and found a cost–benefit ratio of 2.94, meaning that every $1 spent produced $2.94 benefit.

In some instances **discounting** is used for costs over time and for those benefits which emerge in the distant future – that is, an annual percentage reduction can be used to adjust for the declining value of money over time and the presumed lesser value of benefits. There are concerns that this favours interventions which produce outcomes relatively rapidly. Decisions about the discount rate to apply to benefits are also subjective and based on value judgements about immediate as opposed to future gains. Conventionally, the same rate is used for costs and benefits, but because health is seen as different from other commodities lower or even zero rates are generally used. A review of cost-effectiveness studies by the National Institute for Clinical Excellence (NICE 2005) noted that the additional benefit of nicotine replacement therapy over and above brief advice ranged from £350 to £800 per life year gained, based on 1998 prices and using a discount rate of 6 per cent for costs and 1.5 per cent for benefits.

Proponents of economic evaluation contend that the information it can provide is needed to make decisions about how best to allocate resources. Indeed, within a cash-limited service such considerations are held to be required ethically to ensure funds are used to maximum effect. However, critics have argued that faith in economic rationality is misplaced. Concerns about such approaches range from the technical to the philosophical and ethical. The procedures used for economic evaluation of biomedical interventions do not lend themselves easily to public health interventions which, typically, do not fit into a narrow causally determined pathway from inputs to outcomes. Furthermore, it is not merely a question of the need for technical refinement, but of a fundamental mismatch between essentially modernist economic evaluation and the post-modern nature of health promotion and public health practice (Burrows *et al.* 1995).

Godfrey (2001) notes that the principal criterion for economic evaluation is to maximize the outcomes achieved within a given budget. In cost-effectiveness terms, interventions targeted at populations that are relatively 'easy' to change would be favoured in comparison to those targeted at groups more resistant to change or those coping with more adverse social circumstances – ultimately widening health inequalities. Economic efficiency cannot therefore be the sole criterion and has to be considered alongside other goals such as equity, regeneration, social inclusion and social justice.

Burrows *et al.* (1995) express concern that 'discourses – such as health economics – which are strong on "truth claims" may come to dominate decisions. The fundamental question is whether economic considerations are useful and ethical in choices about the competing use of resources. Craig and Walker (1996) reframe the purpose of economic evaluations from the pursuit of economic objectives to identifying and considering the economic consequences of taking different courses of action. This includes the sacrifices, or opportunity costs, incurred by not adopting an alternative course of action. Economic evaluation, from this perspective, can be an aid, but not the sole criterion used, in decision-making (Craig and Walker 1996; Tolley *et al.* 1996).

Godfrey notes that producing accurate cost-effectiveness information is dependent on health promotion and public health taking a rigorous approach to evaluation and generating practical outcome measures which capture the full impact of interventions. She suggests that full economic evaluations are not appropriate in many instances and that they should be used 'wisely, not widely or without the application of other evaluation methods' (Godfrey 2001: 161).

The importance of objectives

When programme goals are expressed with precision, defining what constitutes success should follow naturally. Conversely, when there is little clarity about goals, defining success is more problematic. It has been recognized for some time that poor definition and measurement of outcomes have been a problem for evaluating public health and health promotion interventions:

> Poor definition of programme objectives – whether these are expressed in terms of valued outcomes and/or valued processes – often leads to inappropriate expectations concerning evaluation and accountability. . . . it is essential that programme objectives are more clearly defined, and that relevant and sensitive measures are used to assess progress in achieving these objectives. (Nutbeam 1998: 41)

Valued outcomes, such as empowerment, participation and positive well-being, are particularly challenging to measure compared with disease states or physical function. Nutbeam (1998) has identified three levels of outcomes as a framework for identifying the range of possible intervention outcomes.

- *Health and social outcomes.* Social outcomes constitute the highest level and possibly the ultimate goal for public health and health promotion interventions. They include quality of life, functional independence and equity. Underpinning these are more narrowly defined physical and mental health outcomes which include mortality, morbidity and disability.
- *Intermediate health outcomes.* This level is concerned with the determinants of health and social outcomes. It includes health behaviours, environmental influences (physical, social and economic), and access to and use of services.

- *Health promotion outcomes.* This basic level is concerned with the immediate personal, social and environmental factors that allow people to take control of their health. As such, this level represents the primary focus for many public health interventions and their immediate outcomes. It includes: knowledge, values, attitudes, motivation and skills; social influence and action, including social connectedness, social support, community engagement, community empowerment; and policy and organization practices which support a healthy environment (physical, social and economic).

While aims or goals set out in broad terms what an intervention might achieve, objectives provide a precise definition. The formulation of objectives is central to programme planning and evaluation. The acronym SMART is often used to identify the essentials of a clear objective:

Specific
Measurable
Achievable
Realistic
Time-related

The most rigorous way of constructing objectives is as behavioural objectives which state what the 'learner' is able to do and follow the pattern: who will do/be able to do what, to what extent and when. For example:

People who have completed an exercise on prescription programme will exercise for 30 minutes a day five times a week six months after completion of the programme.

While at first sight this might appear to conform with the pattern, Mager (1975: 21) suggests that objectives should also specify conditions and acceptable levels of performance:

1. *Performance.* An objective always says what a learner is able to do.

2. *Condition.* An objective always describes what the important conditions (if any) are under which the performance is to occur.

3. *Criterion.* Wherever possible, an objective describes the criterion of acceptable performance by describing how well the learner must perform in order to be considered acceptable.

We might therefore rephrase the example as:

50 per cent people who have satisfactorily completed the exercise on prescription programme will report, when asked, taking part in moderate activity for 30 minutes a day at least five times a week, six months after completion of the programme.

Some consideration could also be given to what constitutes satisfactory completion of the programme – attending all sessions or a minimum number? Clearly, specifying a level of achievement is dependent on having appropriate baseline data and an understanding of trends and, as we noted above, this can be problematic.

While, at first sight, it may seem that SMART objectives are more appropriate for individually targeted behaviour change initiatives, they can equally apply to community development and policy initiatives. For example:

> Immediately after a participatory appraisal of needs, residents will report, when asked, that they feel more confident that their views are listened to. Two months after a publicity campaign, 90 per cent of local counsellors will identify accurately, when interviewed, the locality with the highest rate of road injuries.

↻ Points for reflection – SMART objectives

Consider what might be appropriate SMART objectives for the following:

- Smoking cessation clinic
- Legislation to ban smoking in pubs
- Improvement of school lunches

Indicators

Clearly, for most evaluations it is neither feasible nor desirable to measure every possible variable – which we might refer to as the 'If it moves, count it' phenomenon. Instead, indicators are usually selected to capture key aspects of the programme and its effects. There are alternative views about the nature of indicators. Allan *et al.* (2004: 2) note that for some, and particularly in relation to large-scale evaluations, the term is interpreted narrowly as 'a quantitative measure, generated from data collected for administrative purposes, which comprises aggregated data relating to a defined population at a specific point in time'. From this perspective, routinely collected data such as receipt of benefits, unemployment statistics, Standard Assessment Test scores of children's achievement at school, and child injury statistics could potentially be used as indicators of the effectiveness of Sure Start, a government programme targeted at disadvantaged areas which aims to achieve better outcomes for children, parents and communities. However, in the context of public health, this interpretation is overly restrictive in a number of ways. Firstly, it places emphasis on quantitative data and ignores the importance of the qualitative perspective. Secondly, the type of information available may be insufficient to adequately capture the full range of possible outcomes.

Thirdly, routinely collected data is usually aggregated at the area level which may create difficulties if the area targeted by the intervention is not coterminous with the administrative area for which the data is presented. For example, the catchment area for a school could easily include both a Sure Start area and a neighbouring area not served by Sure Start. Any school-based data will therefore be an amalgam of both. Even when this is not the case, aggregation can produce some distortion by overlooking variation between subgroups within the target population.

An alternative broader definition is that indicators are 'specific measures indicating the point at which goals and/or objectives have been achieved. Often they are proxies for goals and objectives which cannot be directly measured' (Health Communication Unit 2006: 19). In short, they identify the information needed to respond to the question 'How will we know if the objectives have been achieved or progress is being made towards achieving them?'. This interpretation would accommodate the use of qualitative indicators. It would also include indicators that require the development of appropriate data-collection systems rather than relying on secondary data.

The fundamental issue is that indicators should be valid and accurately represent what they claim to represent. Absentee rates have been proposed as a possible indicator of pupils' dissatisfaction with school. The rate of absenteeism will be influenced to some extent by the level of satisfaction with the school, but other factors are also involved – not least the rigour of measures to control absenteeism. Even though this data may be readily available, it can be regarded as only loosely indicative of satisfaction. A better indicator may be the views of pupils themselves, which could be obtained using questionnaires or in-depth interviewing. In some instances problems relating to availability of information, measurement and data collection may make it simply not feasible to identify valid indicators. In this situation it may be possible to use proxy indicators. For example, the rate of gonorrhoea is sometimes used as a proxy indicator for all sexually transmitted infection and also for the prevalence of unsafe sexual practices. NHS local delivery plans for sexual health are required to include a target for reducing the rate of gonorrhoea by 2008 (Department of Health 2005a). Allen *et al.* (2004) emphasize the importance of defining the concept for which the proxy measure is to stand in order to ensure that it is relevant. They refer to the use of data on children's oral health as a proxy indicator for children's general health, but question its appropriateness for children's mental health.

Although the pursuit of validity should be the central concern in the selection of indicators, practical feasibility is inevitably also an issue. The danger of allowing this to dominate is aptly conveyed by the MacNamara fallacy (see Box 3.4) which is often summed up as making the measurable important, rather than the important measurable.

Box 3.4 The MacNamara fallacy

The first step is to measure whatever can be easily measured. This is OK as far as it goes.

The second step is to disregard that which can't easily be measured or to give it an arbitrary quantitative value. This is artificial and misleading.

The third step is to presume that what can't be measured easily isn't important. This is blindness.

The fourth step is to say that what can't easily be measured really doesn't exist. This is suicide.

(Handy 1994: 219)

Point for reflection

What are the implications of the MacNamara fallacy for the selection of indicators?

The selection of indicators is ultimately influenced by values. Springett (1998b: 169) contends that 'the process of developing and using indicators to evaluate healthy public policy is more a political problem than a technical one, depending on world views and power structures, including the ability to impose certain opinions on others'. There is a tendency to use indicators of ill-health rather than health, reflecting 'traditional medical norms and managerial outcomes', even when programmes derive from a socio-ecological model of health. Furthermore, the views of target groups about what would be important indicators of success for them are often overlooked, as we will note in Chapter 5.

The identification of appropriate indicators should be relatively straightforward if programme objectives are well defined and comprehensive and espouse all goals and values integral to the programme. SMART objectives should therefore lead to SMART indicators:

Specific
Measurable
Appropriate
Relevant
Time-related

An alternative acronym, SPICED, is also often used to emphasize the need to include qualitative measures and address some of the concerns referred to above. SPICED indicators are:

Subjective
Participatory

Interpretable
Cross-checked
Empowering
Disaggregated
(Allan *et al.* 2004; BOND n.d.)

Points for reflection

At the end of the previous section you were asked to set appropriate SMART objectives for a smoking cessation clinic, legislation to ban smoking in pubs, and improvement of school lunches. Now suggest suitable SMART or SPICED indicators.

Intermediate, outcome and process indicators

We noted above the hierarchy of outcomes identified by Nutbeam. The outcomes of a programme may be considered as a 'succession of often complex and interacting series of temporal events' (Tones 1998: 63). They may be ordered in relation to a time-scale starting with the more *proximal* effects which occur relatively soon followed by progressively later *distal* effects ending with the ultimate strategic goal. This can apply regardless of whether the anticipated outcomes are conceived in terms of the prevention of ill-health or the promotion of positive well-being. For example, the anticipated outcomes of a programme to increase physical activity among a socially deprived group could be arranged in order as follows:

increased awareness of opportunities and motivation to increase physical activity

↓

increase in physical activity

↓

increase in well-being, physiological measures of fitness, improved Body Mass Index

↓

decrease in coronary heart disease, better quality of life

↓

reduction in health inequalities, social justice

For many programmes the focus is on the achievement of more immediate outcomes rather than ultimate strategic goals. **Outcome indicators** need to be framed in terms of the realistic aspirations for a programme. There is frequently pressure to demonstrate reduction in disease using epidemiological indicators. However, this may be neither necessary nor feasible. The crucial question is how far along the causal sequence from intervention to ultimate goal the evaluation needs to go. Where there is already well-established evidence of the link between behavioural outcomes and disease reduction outcomes, there is no need to subject this to further study. Green and Tones (1999) have argued forcefully that such evidence is the justification for implementing the programme in the first place rather than the means of evaluating its effects. All that would be necessary in this instance would be to identify appropriate outcome indicators of behaviour change. The evaluation of the National Healthy School Standard (NHSS) noted the difficulty of measuring health outcomes:

> It is to be hoped that effective health education will lead ultimately to improved health and the reduction of illness, but this is a very long-term prospect. Within the scope of the evaluation, it is unlikely that NHSS activities would have a direct effect on these outcomes. Therefore, we need to focus on health-related behaviour, the intermediate step between health promotion activities and impact on health. (Blenkinsop *et al.* 2004: 52)

Intermediate indicators would occur earlier in the causal sequence and include any of the antecedents of the outcome indicator/s. Whether indicators are classified as outcome or intermediate is to an extent a matter of definition. Indeed, the same variable could be used as an outcome indicator for some programmes and as an intermediate indicator for others. Empowerment could be the outcome of a community development programme or an intermediate indicator in an educational programme to promote safer sex practice among young women. Understanding the anticipated series of stages in the change sequence is fundamental to identifying appropriate indicators. We will look at this in more detail in the discussion of Theory of Change later in this chapter.

Process indicators are used to record key elements of the process of the intervention itself and can contribute to recording the fidelity and quality of the programme. Programme implementation may involve subsidiary activities and quality measures. Indicators may be required to assess the effectiveness of these – for example, pre-testing mass media programmes or assessing the confidence of teachers to deliver a sex education programme to young people following training. Such indicators are referred to as **indirect indicators** as they are not part of the causal sequence from input to outcomes even though they contribute to the intervention itself. The important point of distinction is between means and ends, whether short- or long-term. Allan *et al.* (2004) comment on the complexity of separating process indicators, outcome indicators and systems indicators which assess quality of management and structures. For example, the development of good partnerships, while a process factor, may also be a positive outcome in itself. This is further illustrated in the example in Chapter 4.

While this distinction between different types of indicator can and should be made in very small-scale projects, the use of these various indicators allows the progress of complex national and regional initiatives towards achieving their targets to be tracked. For example, the Tackling Health Inequalities Programme for Action draws on a number of indicator sets. These include:

- PSA [Public Service Agreement] target reports
- national headline indicators
- PPF/LDP [Priorities and Planning Framework/Local Delivery Plan] target indicators
- comprehensive performance assessment
- local basket of indicators. (Department of Health 2005c: 20)

The PSA target is held to be the overall goal of the programme, whereas the national headline indicators (see Box 3.5) are a proxy measure of progress and likely to be the first to pick up outcomes. They offer 'simple, summary snapshots of progress on key interventions, reflecting data already collected' (Department of Health 2005c: 12).

Box 3.5 National headline indicators – Tackling Health Inequalities: The Programme for Action

- Death rates from the big killers – cancer and heart disease
- Teenage conception rate
- Road accident casualty rates in disadvantaged communities
- Numbers of primary care professionals
- Uptake of flu vaccinations
- Smoking among manual groups and among pregnant women
- Educational attainment
- Consumption of fruit and vegetables
- Proportion in non-decent housing
- PE and school sport
- Children in poverty
- Homeless families living in temporary accommodation

(Department of Health 2005c: 12)

Comprehensive performance assessment, in contrast, includes a process element by responding to the key question:

What has the council, with its partners, done to achieve its ambitions for the promotion of healthier communities and the narrowing of health inequalities and are these achievements recognised by the local population? (Department of Health 2005c: 22)

In addition to the national data sets, local progress can be assessed using the local basket of indicators developed by the London Health Observatory (see Box 3.6). Each of the broad sections listed in Box 3.6 is broken down into more detailed indicators with data sources. The Health Poverty Index (see Table 3.3) is a useful visualization tool which allows local authority areas to compare their progress against the national position and again has links to appropriate sources of data from each of the indicators listed.

We emphasized in Chapter 2 that it is not sufficient to merely demonstrate that an input will produce certain outcomes. We need to look inside the

Table 3.3 Health Poverty Index

Root causes	Regional prospects	GDP
		Change in job supply Educational resourcing
	Local conditions	Social capital Education quality
	Household conditions	Income Wealth Human capital
Intervening factors	Resourcing to support health	Local government resourcing Preventative care resourcing
	Healthy areas	Recreation facilities Access to preventative healthcare Quality of preventative healthcare
	Behaviours and environments	Lifestyle Home environments Work and local environments
Situation of health	Resourcing for health and social care	Health care resourcing Social care resourcing
	Appropriate care	Effective primary/secondary care Access to secondary care Access to social care Quality of social care
	Health status	Psychological morbidity Health capital Physical morbidity Premature mortality

Source: Dibben *et al.* (2004).

Box 3.6 Local indicators of inequality

Local basket of indicators

Section 1	Employment, Poverty and Deprivation
Section 2	Housing and Homelessness
Section 3	Education
Section 4	Crime
Section 5	Pollution and Physical Environment
Section 6	Community Development
Section 7	Lifestyle including Diet, Smoking and Physical Activity
Section 8	Access to Local Health and Other Services
Section 9	Accidents and Injury
Section 10	Mental Health
Section 11	Maternal, Infant and Child Health
Section 12	Older People
Section 13	Tackling the Major Killers

'black box' between inputs and outcomes to attempt to understand how change comes about and elucidate the complex relationships between process and outcomes. Using 'realist' terminology (Pawson and Tilley 1997) we need to understand the mechanism of change and how, with reference to contextual factors, it produces outcomes. Clearly the various types of indicator referred to here will be linked through causal chains or webs. We now turn our attention to Theory of Change, which opens the black box to elucidate these linkages (Granger 1998). Conceptually it has similarities with realistic evaluation discussed in Chapter 2, but stakeholders generate the theory or assumptions linking activities with outcomes as an initial stage in the evaluation.

The Theory of Change approach

The Theory of Change approach to evaluation has its origins in the work of Chen, Rossi and Weiss and was further developed in relation to **comprehensive community initiatives** (large, multi-dimensional, community-based programmes, also referred to as **complex community initiatives**) by the Aspen Institute Roundtable on Community Change (Fulbright-Anderson *et al.* 1998). A member of the roundtable, Carol Weiss, suggested that:

> a key reason complex programs are so difficult to evaluate is that the assumptions that inspire them are poorly articulated ... stakeholders of complex community initiatives typically are unclear about how the

change process will unfold and therefore place little attention to the early and mid-term changes that need to happen in order for a longer term goal to be reached. The lack of clarity about the 'mini-steps' that must be taken to reach a long term outcome not only makes the task of evaluating a complex initiative challenging, but reduces the likelihood that all of the important factors related to the long term goal will be addressed. (Aspen Institute n.d.)

Initiatives are often undertaken with only implicit assumptions about how they might work and achieve their goals. The Theory of Change approach centres on surfacing this latent theory.

For many public health and social interventions this relationship is complex. The intervention itself may involve a whole raft of activities targeted at different levels, including the individual, families, communities and organizations – for example healthy schools, healthy living centres, Sure Start Local Programmes. Activities and outcome are connected by an intersecting web rather than a simple linear sequence.

Connell and Kubisch (1998) emphasize that Theory of Change is an approach to evaluation and not a method. Indeed it can draw on many different methods and methodologies. The approach involves setting out the series of outcomes that are expected to unfold as a result of the various components of the intervention as a basis for planning the evaluation strategy. The development of the theory involves a combination of existing knowledge/theory, 'practitioner wisdom' and the insight of local stakeholders through a 'guided process . . . to create a written explicit description of how stakeholders expect to move from activities to their goals' (Granger 1998). They refer to early descriptions of surfacing the theory of change as 'a process in which stakeholders and evaluators "co-construct" the initiative's theory so as to maximize its utility for all'. However, they identify a number of challenges associated with generating the theory and 'reconciling multiple theories of change'. They propose, as a first stage, the identification of longer-term outcomes, as their experience has shown that achieving agreement on these is easiest. Working back from these the intermediate outcomes, contextual factors, activities and the resources needed can be identified (see Box 3.7).

Box 3.7 The stages in the Theory of Change approach to evaluation

- Identifying long-term goals and the assumptions behind them.
- Backwards mapping [to] connect the preconditions or requirements necessary to achieve that goal.
- Identifying the interventions that [the] initiative will perform to create [the] desired change.

- Developing indicators to measure [the] outcomes to assess the performance of [the] initiative.
- Writing a narrative to explain the logic of [the] initiative. (ActKnowledge and Aspen Institute Roundtable on Community Change n.d.)

↻ **Point for reflection**

Consider what the various stages might be in a programme to reduce teen pregnancy rates.

Connell and Kubisch (1998) suggest that the characteristics of a good theory of change are that it is:

- plausible
- doable
- testable.

Different stakeholders may well have different views about important outcomes and how they might be achieved deriving from their own theory of change. However, provided they are not contradictory, it may be possible to accommodate these different views. They key point is that they are articulated:

> The requirements that theories be articulated and that they be specific enough for stakeholders to make judgments about whether or not they are plausible, doable, and testable do not preclude those theories from incorporating multiple perspectives on what long-term outcomes are important, what the interim steps are to getting to those long-term outcomes, and what activities should be implemented. (Connell and Kubisch 1998).

Once the theory of change has been articulated and agreed to be plausible by the stakeholders, it is made testable by identifying appropriate measures and indicators for achievement of the various stages. Emergent patterns in the data are identified and linked back to presumed cause. The 'theory of change approach contends that the more the events predicted by the theory actually occur over the course of [a comprehensive community initiative], the more confidence evaluators and others should have that the initiative's theory is right' (Connell and Kubisch 1998). In the absence of any other 'obvious and pervasive contextual shift' that could have accounted for the change, it is reasonable to attribute it to the intervention. However, Theory of Change 'cannot eliminate all alternative explanations for a particular outcome' (Judge and Bauld 2001: 25). Granger (1998) proposes three strategies to increase the trustworthiness of causal inferences:

- creatively blending designs to create reasonably strong counterfactuals
- explicating and testing for patterns within and across sites and time

- investigating possible causes and effects using mixed data-collection methods and modes of analysis.

Connell and Kubisch (1998) identify three main benefits for starting evaluation with consideration of the theory of change:

1 It can sharpen the planning and implementation of an initiative.
2 It can facilitate the identification of data requirements.
3 Articulating a theory of change which is agreed by all stakeholders can reduce the problem of causal attribution.

The Theory of Change approach was used in the national evaluation of the Health Action Zones (HAZs) in England (Judge 2000). HAZs were set up in 1998 as complex, partnership-based initiatives to tackle health inequalities and social exclusion by improving the health and well-being of the most disadvantaged groups. Judge and Bauld (2001: 21) note that 'Only in very rare cases was it possible at the outset to identify a clear and logical pathway that linked problems, strategies for intervention, milestones or targets with associated time scales and longer term outcomes or goals'. They make three key points about the development of the theory. First, they are not simple but multi-layered. Second, implementation theory, which is concerned with how an intervention is implemented, should be distinguished from programmatic theory, which focuses on how activities achieve change. Third, the theory of change should be sufficiently clear to allow stakeholders to agree the following key requirements for monitoring and evaluation:

> Indicators: which indicators will demonstrate that a particular element's outcomes are changing?
>
> Populations: which target populations should be showing change on these indicators?
>
> Thresholds: how much change on these indicators is good enough?
>
> Timelines: how long will it take to achieve these thresholds?
>
> (Judge and Bauld 2001: 27)

They emphasize that indicators should be specified in advance and be consistent with the articulated theory of change, and that it should be relatively easy to assess whether the predicted steps in the sequence of change have been achieved. The practical application of Theory of Change will be considered more fully in Chapter 5.

Mackenzie and Blamey's (2005) analysis of the experience of using Theory of Change to evaluate comprehensive community initiatives in Scotland identifies a number of challenges which resonate with the experience of the English HAZs. Although, in an ideal situation, the theory of change should be articulated at the planning stage, the practical reality in the case of external evaluations is that evaluation teams and programme teams often come together much later. Further, the pressure to get projects up and running means that they are often well under way before this takes place.

Mackenzie and Blamey found the greatest difficulty in getting projects to identify outcomes that were sufficiently specific to measure progress – particularly quantifiable measures and the expected magnitude of change. They suggest: 'There may have been a blame culture in many of these organizations and so asking implementers to prospectively set targets (particularly challenging targets) may have been viewed as a stick to "beat their backs with"' (Mackenzie and Blamey 2005: 161). Notwithstanding these difficulties and the length of the process, Mackenzie and Blamey concluded that the use of Theory of Change met the claims noted above that this approach can improve planning and provide a focus for evaluation. However, they were less convinced about claims for addressing problems of attribution.

Logic models

It has been noted that the Theory of Change approach does not provide tools for actually unpacking and identifying the theory of change. Logical frameworks have been used to achieve more effective programme planning and are also a useful device for checking the assumptive logic underpinning programme development (Nancholas 1998). They also enable indicators to be identified. The Logframe matrix or logical framework is made up of a 4×4 matrix as shown in Table 3.4.

Table 3.4 A Logframe matrix

	Narrative summary	Verifiable indicators	Means of verification	Assumptions
Goal Why are we doing this?				
Purpose What will we achieve?				
Outputs What immediate outcomes will we achieve?				
Activities What will we do?				

The process of constructing a Logframe is consistent with the Theory of Change approach and involves the active participation of key stakeholders. The goal is usually stated in broad terms – for example, reducing road injuries among children. The purpose of the programme is then specified and should make a direct contribution to the overall goal. Continuing with our example, this could be improving young people's road crossing behaviour or alternatively improving driver behaviour in built-up areas or, in a comprehensive programme, both. However, each Logframe should contain only one goal and one purpose, so in complex initiatives a separate Logframe will have to be completed for each purpose. The outputs are then identified. The term is used in this context to refer to all the immediate results or deliverables of the programme and would include materials and organizational or policy change as well as any behavioural or environmental change. The activities needed to achieve these are then specified. The vertical logic can be verified by working through the stages to check whether, in principle, if each is put in place then the next will logically follow – see Figure 3.2 for a simple worked example.

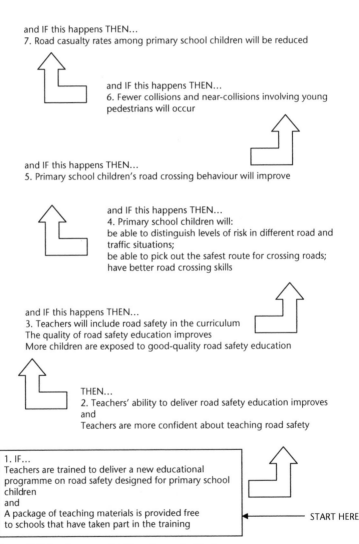

Figure 3.2 Logframes – checking the vertical logic

This process will make explicit any assumption at each level and enable the theory of change to be developed. It will provide a check that all necessary conditions are in place to achieve the overall goal and expose any potentially fatal flaws in the design. In the case of Figure 3.2 there is an assumption that safe places to cross exist. Moreover, focusing on child behaviour ignores the contribution of road design and driver behaviour to child pedestrian injury, an example we will take up in Chapter 4.

Objectively verifiable indicators (OVIs) are developed for each stage in the vertical hierarchy and the means of verification (MOV) identified. Returning to our example, possible OVIs and MOV for selected outcomes are shown in Table 3.5.

Table 3.5 Identification of indicators and means of verification

	OVI	MOV
Outcome 3		
Teachers will include road safety in the curriculum	Amount of time allocated to road safety in the curriculum	Questionnaire to schools
The quality of road safety education improves	Quality assessment of teaching	Observation of teaching Questionnaire including quality criteria for assessing teaching
More children are exposed to good-quality road safety education	Numbers of children receiving road safety education at school	Questionnaire for school staff Focus-group discussions with pupils on quality of road safety education
Outcome 4		
Primary school children will: be able to distinguish levels of risk in different road and traffic situations;	Ability to distinguish levels of risk associated with different crossing situations	No. of pupils correctly placing pictures showing different scenarios in order of risk No. of pupils who can correctly identify hazards in photographs of real traffic situations
be able to pick out the safest route for crossing roads;		No. of pupils correctly identifying safe routes in a range of simulations Observation of children's road crossing behaviour in real-life situations
have better road crossing skills		Observation of children crossing roads in a simulation and in real-life situations

Daniel and Dearden (2001) identified a number of advantages of using Logframes in planning HAZ Innovation Fund projects:

- systematic, logical and thorough
- imposes discipline and structure
- identifies risks and assumptions
- provides a framework for monitoring and evaluation
- encourages the development of partnerships
- provides flexibility and adaptability.

The use of logical frameworks is not restricted to major demonstration projects, but is equally relevant for small-scale local projects. One person, commenting on their experience of using Logframes, noted:

> Logframes really do take the misery out of project planning for local people, they are simple and clear. The problem for professionals is that [working with Logframes] they have to be transparent – something we have all learnt not to be in order to survive in bureaucracies! Managing the change is the biggest issue, not necessarily managing the Logframe process. (Daniel and Dearden 2001: 6)

Gathering information

A key consideration in the collection of data is whether such information is 'fit for purpose' (Allan *et al.* 2004). The fundamental issue is whether the data is **necessary** to respond to the evaluation questions and whether it is **sufficient** in itself or would require supplementation in some way. In some instances the evaluation may be able to use already existing information. Myers *et al.* (2004) provide detailed guidance on the use of existing data in the context of Sure Start local evaluations and outline the benefits as:

- being less costly than new data collection
- limiting the reporting burden placed on project staff, parents and target groups, reducing the potential for evaluation fatigue
- identification of areas that would benefit from further evaluative study
- rapid identification of gaps in service provision to pinpoint areas for more in-depth study
- providing validation for evaluation findings generated by primary data-collection methods.

Existing information takes a number of forms. It includes data routinely collected and held by the programme and data collected and held by other agencies. Official data may be publicly available, such as ONS Neighbourhood Statistics or accessed through other agencies, such as primary care trusts or local authorities. Key considerations in obtaining data are:

- Who collects it?
- Who collates it?
- Over what area or time period is it aggregated?

- What access is there to the raw or aggregated data?

The National Healthy School Standard evaluation (Blenkinsop *et al.* 2004), mentioned above, provides some insight into the way data sources for the agreed indicators were identified. After consideration of a range of possible data sources, a number were rejected for the following main reasons:

- data was aggregated over areas not coterminous with the area of interest (for example, primary care trust or strategic health authority rather than local education authority)
- problems in gaining access
- unsuitable reporting times.

Blenkinsop *et al.* (2004) also noted that they were unable to locate data sources for two of their agreed indicators. These were age at first sexual intercourse and use of contraception, and instead they explored the use of other indicators of sexual health.

If data is aggregated it will not be possible to identify individuals, whereas other data sets may contain personally identifiable information. Access to the former is clearly easier as it is not subject to the same ethical constraints or the requirements of the Data Protection Act which apply to personal information. This issue is addressed in Chapter 6.

Much data will be collected at the programme level. Drawing on our earlier example of road safety education, Table 3.6 illustrates how monitoring data might be used.

Table 3.6 The use of monitoring data

Source	Type of data	Use
Database	Reach data	Number of schools contacted How many teachers have been trained to deliver the programme Characteristics of schools reached and not reached
Questionnaire to schools	Number of schools using the programme with pupils (uptake)	Proportion of young people reached by the programme in an area
Questionnaire to schools	Amount of curriculum time devoted to the programme	Indicator of programme intensity

Williams and Wright (1998) refer to Murphy's Law of information (see Box 3.8) in relation to the difficulties of obtaining appropriate data for health needs assessment. This might equally apply to evaluation.

Box 3.8 Murphy's Law of information (Williams and Wright 1998)

The information we have is not what we want.
The information we want is not what we need.
The information we need is too expensive to collect.
(Williams and Wright 1998)

Clearly due regard will need to be given to feasibility during the process of defining indicators to ensure that data collection is possible within the evaluation resources. It is essential, at the outset, to identify what data will be routinely available and what will require specific data-collection methods to be set up. Similarly, the respective responsibilities of the project and evaluation teams for data collection will need to be clarified where evaluation is undertaken in partnership. Co-research involving an external evaluator and the project team is potentially advantageous in that it 'prioritises a direct relationship between evaluator and [project] and it seeks to develop the research framework through a process of exchange between the two' (Sullivan *et al.* 2002: 222).

It is beyond the scope of this text to discuss data-collection methods in detail, and there are numerous specialist texts on research methods. To an extent, the indicators selected will prescribe the data-collection methods required. Over and above the use of secondary data, primary data-collection methods such as questionnaires of various types, structured and in-depth interviews and focus groups may be needed.

A key criterion in selecting methods and developing data-collection instruments is the issue of reliability and validity. **Reliability** refers to the capacity of the research methods to consistently generate the same findings when recording the same situation. **Validity** concerns the extent to which the methods and process of data collection actually measure what they set out to measure. We noted above the need for conceptual clarity in defining indicators. Judge and Bauld (2001: 20) advise that 'mixed methods and the careful triangulation of evidence offer the best way forward in learning about complex initiatives'. **Internal validity** is the capacity of an evaluation to demonstrate whether an intervention had achieved the outcomes identified and, hence, includes both the accurate measurement and attribution of change. **External validity** allows inferences to be made for other groups from the findings. From a positivist perspective this might involve ensuring that the study population is representative of the wider population. However, the realist evaluation position would be that the findings of a particular context-specific evaluation cannot be transferred piecemeal to another situation. Rather, the emphasis should be on elucidating the specific context and the way it interacts with the mechanism of change to achieve outcomes as a basis for understanding what might work elsewhere.

A further consideration in the selection of data-collection methods is that they are suitable for the various respondent groups. For instance, the evaluation of interventions targeted at young children may need to draw on methods appropriate for this age group. Draw and write methods have been widely used in health research with children, although the method is not without its critics (Pridmore 1996; Backett-Milburn and McKie 1999). Clearly it is important that data collection does not just focus on the views of those who are easily reached and attempts to avoid **chatty bias** – 'A general problem which arises when the views of more outspoken individuals (e.g. experts) tend to stand out, although their views may not be representative' (UK Evaluation Society 2003a). This would equally apply to the more vocal members of communities and organizations. If the perspective of difficult-to-reach or marginalized groups is to be included within the evaluation then attention will need to be given to this in the selection and possible adaptation of methods – an issue we will consider more fully in Chapter 7. Furthermore, evaluation methods should reflect the intervention's overall philosophy and approach. If an intervention is participatory, it would be inconsistent to adopt evaluation methods which are essentially 'top down'. For example, the methods used in a small-scale evaluation of a youth work project listed in Box 3.9 were selected on account of the fact that they are participatory and similar to the activities used by the project itself.

Box 3.9 Methods used in the evaluation of the Bingley Young People's Health Project (Green and Newell 2003)

- Question and answer sheets (completed individually) included both closed and open questions.
- Completion of sentence stems on graffiti sheets. Sentence stems used to trigger responses included 'The best things about BYPHP . . .', 'The worst things about BYPHP . . .', 'Things I would change and how . . .'.
- Focus-group discussion to encourage participation, reflect on the collective experience and help trigger and organize ideas.
- Video interviewing. Young people were put into the role of television news crews with the task of developing an interview 'script' to find out issues they considered to be important. They then used this to interview and record other group members.

Points for reflection

What methods might be appropriate to assess the provision of play and learning opportunities for children in an area for use with:

- parents/carers?
- children?

As we have already noted, indicators of process and programme implementation are needed as well as outcomes. Frequently such information focuses on:

> the technology of the intervention without informing us about how the context in which it was implemented affected the technology. We learn little about the many compromises, choice points and backroom conversations that allowed it to take the form it took. (Trickett 1998: 329, cited in Riley and Hawe 2005)

Methods will need to address the complexity of implementation – for example, narrative methods, which we will discuss more fully in Chapter 8.

Summary

In this chapter we have considered the issue of success and have noted the importance of clear objectives in defining success and establishing appropriate indicators. Unpacking anticipated change pathways allows outcomes to be ordered in a time sequence and a range of indicators identified from early (proximal) to late (distal). The use of Theory of Change and logic models can help to clarify goals, change pathways, identify indicators and reach a consensus among the key stakeholder groups. Having a clear view of outcomes and precision in developing indicators facilitates the collection of appropriate information and the capacity to 'capture' change. At the same time it should not 'blinker' the evaluator to any unanticipated outcomes – either positive or negative. We have emphasized the importance of process and the need to develop process indicators.

The selection of methods for measuring outcomes and process should be based on consideration of reliability, validity, suitability for purpose, feasibility, consistency with the values and methods of working of the project and appropriateness for use with various groups.

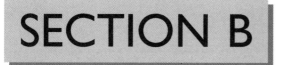

SECTION B

Practice

4 Developing an evaluation plan

Overview

This chapter is about putting principles into practice and deals with the practicalities of designing and managing an evaluation. The chapter includes:

- a simple evaluation framework in six steps
- issues to consider when commissioning and planning an evaluation
- guidance on setting up data-collection systems
- a worked example of an evaluation plan
- suggested resources for evaluation in practice.

Evaluation planning

Like any activity, evaluation benefits from being well planned. A structured approach to collecting and interpreting evidence is required, whether it is a large programme or a small-scale project, so that questions such as 'Is this initiative effective?' and 'How and why does it work?' can be answered satisfactorily. WHO Guidance on Evaluating Health Promotion (Springett 1998a) suggests that evaluation should be seen as an iterative process with each stage based on a cycle of **reflection**, **planning**, **action** and **change**. This enables transparency about choices from the start through to the finish of the project. Having examined the general principles of evaluation and discussed some of the contrasting theories and approaches in Chapters 2 and 3, we now turn to the practicalities of designing and managing an evaluation. The purpose of this chapter is to set out key areas for consideration in developing a robust evaluation plan with the focus on undertaking small-scale evaluations. Readers are provided with a simple evaluation framework in the form of a series of six steps. Inevitably we revisit some of the principles of evaluation in looking at their application to practice.

Evaluation planning is the process of clarifying what needs to be researched and identifying how evidence will be collected. Rushing in and collecting data in an *ad hoc* fashion, or alternatively researching everything that moves in the hope that something significant will emerge, will not result in meaningful conclusions being drawn and is ultimately a waste of resources. In contrast, developing a plan can help those involved in an evaluation to steer a path through the mass of information about a programme. A good evaluation plan will:

- clarify the programme objectives and develop understanding of how programme activities contribute to goals;
- allow appropriate indicators and research methods to be chosen;
- identify sources of evidence and also gaps where evidence is not available;
- identify priorities for data collection;
- provide a framework for the interpretation of data;
- help managers allocate adequate and appropriate resources for evaluation.

Preliminary considerations

In the early stages of planning there are a number of considerations. Where evaluations are commissioned, those responsible will confirm the focus of the evaluation, the time-scale and available funding prior to awarding contracts. Even where evaluation is done internally by practitioners, there needs to be an allocation of resources and delineation of responsibilities. Evaluability assessment offers a planning framework where agreement is sought with stakeholders (Thurston and Potvin 2003). St Leger *et al.* (1992) suggest that a protocol is drawn up and responsibilities clarified for four aspects of the evaluation process: commissioning; overseeing; doing; supporting and enabling. Small steering groups can be convened with the purpose of defining evaluation priorities and agreeing management and reporting mechanisms.

Decisions about the scope of the evaluation need to be made. Agreeing the primary purpose of an evaluation will guide choices in terms of design and approach. An evaluation that is commissioned primarily as a demonstration project will require a different approach and level of resources than an evaluation undertaken with the purpose of informing the future direction of a project. Whether the focus is primarily on outcomes or processes or a mixture of both is another consideration (Nutbeam 1998; Wright 1999). The evaluation framework of the Health Education Board for Scotland (HEBS) (see Table 4.1) provides a useful categorization of stages of programme development and the type of evaluation required (Wimbush and Watson 2000; HEBS n.d.). As discussed earlier, because of the difficulties in distinguishing impact and outcome and different interpretations in general use, in this book we use 'outcome evaluation' to refer to the assessment of short-, intermediate- and long-term outcomes.

Clarity is needed about the subject of the evaluation and the boundaries of the investigation (Øvretveit 1998). While it might be obvious who and what is included in small discrete projects, defining boundaries can be more problematical in complex programmes, or where projects have evolved over time. If necessary criteria can be agreed in relation to:

- geographical boundaries
- programme activities

Table 4.1 Stages of project development and evaluation (from HEBS Evaluation Framework)

Stage of project development	Type of evaluation	Purpose of evaluation
Planning	Systematic reviews	Overview of evidence of effectiveness from outcome evaluations
Design and pilot	Developmental evaluation	To assess the feasibility, practicability and acceptability of a project and its processes/mechanisms To test the potential effectiveness of a new approach
Implementation – early start up	Monitoring and review	To monitor and review progress in achieving milestones and agreed quality standards
Implementation – establishment	Impact evaluation	To assess the short-term effectiveness of a project in terms of its reach and immediate impacts
Implementation – fully operational	Outcome evaluation	To assess the longer-term effectiveness of a project using intermediate outcome measures
Dissemination	Transfer evaluation	To assess the replicability of a project's mechanisms, processes and outcomes

Source: Wimbush and Watson (2000: 312–13).

- organizational structures
- the role of partner organizations
- participants or target communities.

The evaluation planning framework that now follows is based on a series of six steps:

1 Clarifying aims and objectives
2 Choosing indicators
3 Linking outcomes, indicators and methods
4 Understanding context and process
5 Setting up data-collection systems
6 Bringing it all together.

The framework has been used successfully by the authors for evaluating projects undertaken within public health practice. In our worked example at the end of the chapter, we demonstrate how a plan linking outcomes, indicators and methods can be set out. There are alternative frameworks available, many of which follow similar steps (see Box 4.1 for some suggested resources).

Box 4.1 Resources for evaluation

HEBS Research & Evaluation Toolbox (HEBS n.d.)
Monitoring & Evaluation: Some Tools, Methods & Approaches (World Bank 2004)
Practical Guidance on Evaluating Health Promotion (Springett 1998a)
Evaluating Health Promotion Programs (Health Communication Unit 2006)
An Evaluation Resource for Healthy Living Centres (Meyrick and Sinkler 1999)
Planning and Doing Programme Evaluation: An Introductory Guide for Health Promotion (Waa et al. 1998)
Partnerships for Learning. A Guide to Evaluating Arts Education Projects (Woolf 2004)
The Evaluation Journey. An Evaluation Resource for Community Groups. (McKie et al. 2002)
A Rough Guide to Learning for Healthy Communities through Evaluation (Community Development and Health Network n.d.)
Community Tool Box. Part J. Evaluating Community Programs and Initiatives (University of Kansas n.d.)

Step 1. Clarifying aims and objectives

Clear objectives are the foundation for a good evaluation plan. It is important that those evaluating a programme understand what it is designed to achieve and what success would mean. It is then possible to select measures of success (Stage 2) and choose appropriate data-collection methods (Stage 3). Interpretations of success vary and will fundamentally influence evaluation choices. For example, in two community sports projects working with young people, one project might have objectives around increasing community cohesion and creating positive role models for young people. In contrast, the other project might be trying to achieve increased awareness of the benefits of physical activity. The evaluation plans of the two projects would differ because they would be attempting to measure different things.

The start of evaluation planning is therefore to clarify what the objectives are. Objective setting is a fundamental stage in systematic approaches to planning (Tones and Green 2004), but in practice objectives can fall short of the gold standard and frequently lack specificity (Phillips *et al.* 1994). In addition, current terminology around goals, targets, objectives and quality standards can add confusion as the terms are used in different ways in different contexts. Essentially the evaluator is aiming to understand:

- the overall aims and goals;
- values and underlying approach taken;
- the intermediate and short-term objectives;
- how the activities contribute to meeting the objectives.

It is sometimes helpful for programmes to map their objectives against national or local health targets. Notwithstanding the difficulties of attributing changes in health status to specific activities, there should be an understanding of the contribution made to long-term goals. As we discussed earlier in the book, Theory of Change and Logframe planning are both approaches which seek to unpack the assumptions behind actions and link the steps to achieving goals. While some find these approaches cumbersome, they can be an aid in evaluation planning, and can lead to greater understanding of the logic of programmes (Learmonth and Mackie 2000; Goodstadt *et al.* 2001).

Two common problems occur at this stage which can be dealt with using similar approaches. The first problem is where objectives are implicit and not documented. This is more likely to happen with services and long-standing projects: a sexual health clinic might have explicit objectives around access to contraceptives but aspects such as addressing individual needs will be taken for granted. It is important that evaluators are able to tease out the implicit objectives and gain an understanding of underlying values. The second problem occurs when there is a gap between documented objectives and current understandings, or even when there are conflicting or inconsistent objectives (Øvretveit 1998). The evaluator can address these two problems at the beginning of the evaluation by bringing stakeholders together to articulate what they are trying to achieve. An alternative approach is to use the evaluation to tease out understandings and help develop a rich description of the programme. It is important, however, not to miss any drift in objectives and to be able to distinguish those changes occurring as natural developments of the project and those which indicate there may have been barriers to implementation.

Step 2. Choosing indicators

Once the objectives have been clarified, the next stage is to choose the **indicators of success**. These are simply the measures selected to show whether a programme is achieving what it set out to achieve. Having good, clear objectives in place will make the job of selecting indicators much easier because the elements and direction of a programme are made transparent.

The most logical way to approach the selection of indicators of success is to identify the **expected outcomes**. The objectives and the expected outcomes should match, especially if the objectives have been defined with a high degree of precision. It is a good discipline to think about the key questions: 'What changes will happen?' and 'What difference will the programme make?'. This moves the evaluator away from describing what a programme does or simply counting outputs to really questioning what happens because of the work.

In choosing indicators of success, the evaluator needs to be aware of the theoretical debates around defining success in public health and health promotion, as discussed earlier. For small-scale evaluations, the evaluator is frequently only able to measure the short-term and intermediate (or medium-term) outcomes. In those situations what is needed is an understanding of how short- and medium-term outcomes contribute to long-term health goals (Hepworth 1997; Nutbeam 1998).

Once expected outcomes have been identified, indicators of success can be selected. Indicators can come in a variety of forms but they need to be measurable, in the sense that evidence can be collected on them. Ultimately it is a case of adopting a common-sense approach and choosing aspects that can be measured practically and will provide acceptable evidence that objectives have been met. Sources of indicators include:

- *Research literature*. Looking at how other researchers have evaluated interventions may provide clues as to what indicators can be used and their limitations.
- *Theoretical analyses*. Using theory to unpick key constructs as a useful basis for identifying indicators. This is explained further in Chapter 8.
- *Sets of indicators*. Development work in key fields of work can be a source of inspiration and often provides access to sets of indicators – for example, inequality indicators (Box 8.1).
- *Policy documents*. Many public health initiatives are working within policy frameworks which provide guidance on evaluation including indicators of success and quality criteria.
- *Knowledge of practice*. Indicators can emerge from understandings of what constitutes good and effective practice. Based on their study of evaluation in practice, Learmonth and Mackie (2000) propose that health promotion practitioners should set appropriate quality criteria for evaluation of interventions.
- *Stakeholders*. Project participants, staff and the wider community can be involved in defining criteria for success (Phillips *et al.* 1994; Riley and Riley 1998; Springett 1998a). This 'bottom up' approach to selecting indicators can prove very useful and is discussed further in Chapter 5.

Some outcomes will be very difficult to capture, and in those cases the most relevant and practical indicators should be selected. Bodart and Sapirie (1998: 305) explain: 'An indicator does not describe a situation in its entirety; it may only suggest what a situation is or give a clue to an unmeasurable phenomenon'. For example, we cannot expect to measure whether young men attending a sexual health outreach service actually use the condoms they are given – even reported use may be too sensitive. What we could measure is intention to use or perceptions of risk. In evaluation we are often in the position of using indicators that only measure something indirectly; what is important is that we acknowledge the limitations of chosen measures when the evaluation findings are reported.

Step 3. Linking outcomes, indicators and methods

This part of the framework is about choosing an appropriate design and research methods to collect evidence on the success of a programme. What the evaluator is aiming for is a good fit between each of the indicators of success and the research methods used to gather evidence. A table is a useful means of ensuring that outcomes, indicators and methods are linked, as illustrated in the worked example below. It is at this stage that the plan often comes together and those involved feel there is a clear path identifying what data will be collected and how.

The selection of methods will be informed by understandings of methodology and the strengths and limitations of the different research traditions. Scott (1998) argues that evaluators cannot divorce themselves from these debates. However, decisions on the ground are more often driven by pragmatism and a flexible approach is taken to selection of methods. As we have noted, there is considerable weight behind the argument that evaluation of public health and health promotion interventions requires use of both qualitative and quantitative methods (for example Baum 1995; MacDonald 1996; Coombes 2000). In planning an evaluation, there should be a good justification for combining methods. Milburn *et al.* (1995) identify four different purposes:

- to select the most appropriate methods;
- to illuminate some aspect in more depth;
- to achieve saturation, thereby strengthening evidence;
- to get diversification in terms of different perspectives on the issue.

Selecting methods is much more than simply deciding between quantitative and qualitative methods. Evaluators have at their fingertips a whole menu of possibilities, from the commonplace to the more unusual. Each research method has strengths and limitations and may be more or less suitable in different contexts. The resources provided by Woolf (1999, 2004) and Health Communication Unit (2002) both identify the advantages and disadvantages of a range of methods for evaluation. Patton (1987) suggests that it is helpful to consider the relative merits of achieving depth or breadth of data collection; the evaluator has to achieve an appropriate balance depending on the nature of the evaluation. For example, in evaluating an exercise-on-prescription scheme, a small sample of participants may be interviewed. While this would provide some in-depth data on individuals using the scheme and how it impacted on their health, it would undoubtedly be of value to additionally collect data on referral, utilization and progression from all scheme participants.

When trying to identify potential methods it can be useful to think of what evidence could be collected as part of routine activities and what needs to be collected at specific points in time, by asking questions or by observation.

C̃ **Points for reflection**

What research methods could be used to provide an in-depth understanding of the impact of a healthy eating programme? What particular insights would these methods offer? What factors would influence your choice of methods?

While questionnaires and interviews are commonly used methods, they should only be chosen because they provide the right evidence, not because they are the default option. The final choice of methods will be influenced by a number of factors relating to theoretical, contextual and practical concerns, including:

- *The purpose of the evaluation and requirements for types of evidence.*
- *The nature of the project.* Research methods should fit with the values and ethos of the project and not undermine them (Springett 2001a).
- *Participants and the target population.* Consideration should be given to the acceptability and appropriateness of different methods with different groups of people.
- *Ethical considerations.* Ethical issues may influence choice of approaches, particularly where sensitive issues are being explored through the evaluation.
- *Practical issues.* Choice of methods will be guided by feasibility, coverage, availability of resources and experience of those undertaking the evaluation.

Evaluations will often use a number of different methods to assess effectiveness and understand process. While there should be a link between each indicator and a method of data collection, in practical terms there needs to be some consideration of the whole evaluation. Methods may be chosen because they can be used to measure more than one indicator – for example, a focus group can explore a range of aspects relating to a topic.

Design issues

So far in this section we have ignored the issue of design, which of course dominates the theoretical debates. This is partly because choices over indicators and methods are required whether it is an illuminative evaluation or a randomized controlled trial. For most small- and medium-scale evaluations undertaken in practice, experimental designs are not feasible. Notwithstanding their limited relevance for this scale of project, it is important to be aware of choices over evaluation design. Although there has been a strong critique of the sole use of experimental designs in public health and health promotion (MacDonald 1996; Barreto 2005); they are still an option where there is a need for strong evidence of effectiveness and in those rare situations where it is possible to control for external factors (Wellings and MacDowall 2000).

Most small-scale evaluations undertaken in practice will use non-experimental designs. In planning the design and data-collection methods, the evaluator needs to take into account whether an element of comparison is needed, over time or between different groups. Another factor to consider is ensuring that the design and methods are flexible enough to capture any unanticipated outcomes. Ultimately the choice of design must be a pragmatic one. Thompson (1992: S71) suggests that the evaluator can 'focus on simple, practical, feasible evaluations with research designs that are adequate for obtaining answers to relevant questions'.

Step 4. Understanding context and process

Steps 1–3 focus on collecting evidence to judge the success of a programme in meeting its objectives. In Step 4 consideration is given to how to investigate contextual influences and develop an understanding of the processes. There are a number of reasons for planning to collect data on **process** and **context**. As we have already shown, investigating processes gives an insight into how and why a project has or has not worked. It is important to know if a project has been implemented as planned and is functioning as intended before appropriate judgements can be made in terms of its success (Speller *et al.* 1997; Wright 1999). Appropriate judgements will also depend on having information on the impact of contextual factors. Finally, process evaluation can identify lessons learnt during the project and can highlight elements of good practice (Fawcett *et al.* 2001; Springett 2001a).

In developing an evaluation plan, evaluators have to decide how to investigate context and process and how those findings will be integrated with evidence on outcomes. It is possible, although not advisable, that process evaluation will be done as a completely separate element. In reality, for most small-scale projects, evaluation of process and outcomes takes place together. This has distinct advantages as it is easier to interpret findings and pull out key lessons which are of direct use to practitioners. Even where experimental designs are used, there is justification for undertaking some process evaluation (Parry-Langdon *et al.* 2003).

Process evaluation can generate a huge volume of data and there is a need to be clear about information needs and priorities for data collection. Once these have been identified, then appropriate data-collection methods can be selected. Often methods used to assess outcomes can be extended to also collect data on process. For example, a questionnaire looking at the impact of a training programme could include some questions on satisfaction and acceptability of the method of delivery. Although different methods can be used, Parry-Langdon *et al.* (2003) argue strongly for the use of qualitative interviews in order to discover the full range of experiences and issues.

As a starting point, most evaluations will need to examine the development and delivery of the project and any influencing factors. Evaluators should also question whether there is a need for more in-depth data collection on specific aspects. Many public health initiatives are based on partnership working, and it can be useful to examine the extent and quality of partnership working as part of the evaluation. Other aspects for investigation might include levels of recruitment and participation within a programme and the acceptability of the methods to different stakeholder groups. It is sometimes difficult to differentiate between process and outcomes, especially where short-term objectives are being evaluated. For example, is developing a post-natal support group an outcome or part of the process of establishing support mechanisms to enable outcomes on breastfeeding to be achieved? Potvin *et al.* (2001) suggest that making artificial distinctions between the two is not helpful, but what is required is clarity over the evidence.

Step 5. Setting up data-collection systems

Once the framework has been completed, the evaluator will need to decide when evidence is gathered, by whom and what resources are needed. Ideally systems should be put in place to ensure that data collection is as efficient as possible. By thinking through a number of questions data collection can be streamlined, thereby reducing the burden on projects.

The first two questions to consider are what data have already been collected and what additional data-collection systems need to be put in place. A great deal of evidence can be assembled through routine activities, ranging from documentary material, completion of records, diaries, attendance figures and so on. Where data can be collected as part of routine activity this represents good use of resources, but the evaluator needs to consider what capacity there is to collect data alongside normal practice. Like all data collection, it should be carried out in a systematic way with some attention to criteria for selection and the quality and consistency of recording. Where data are not collected routinely, decisions need to be made about the timing of the data collection.

As well as collection of primary data, it is useful to consider if secondary data sources can be used as evidence. Table 4.2 lists some of the advantages and the drawbacks of using routine data sets for evaluation. Where there are good reasons for utilizing existing data sources, there may still be barriers to gaining access to data. Despite the increase in partnership working, it is often difficult to obtain comparable data as systems, boundaries and categorization differ between agencies. For readers interested in these issues, Myers *et al.* (2004) provide a very useful guide to using existing data which addresses some of the practical issues faced by evaluators.

Table 4.2 Advantages and limitations of using routine data sets for evaluation

Advantages	Limitations
Low cost	Lack of specificity to evaluation questions
Comprehensiveness of collected data sources	Difficulty in identifying target population
Opportunities for comparison	Lack of sensitivity to changes
Opportunities for analysis of trends over time	Difficulty in inferring causality
Objectivity	Data quality (accuracy, completeness and currency)
	Time-frame of the evaluation

Source: Kane *et al.* (2000).

The next question to consider is who will collect the data. Part of the evaluation planning process should involve clarifying who will be involved in data collection and what their responsibilities are. The lead evaluator will identify the resources that are needed to undertake the data collection and whether extra training or support is required. One key question for managers is the ease with which a practitioner can incorporate data collection into his or her role.

Other questions which can be asked are when data should be collected and whether there is a need to collect baseline data in order to measure changes in key indicators. The choice of evaluation design will dictate, to some extent, the use of pre- and post-tests. In non-experimental designs, whether baseline data can sensibly be collected depends on the nature of what is being evaluated and the stage at which the evaluation is planned. It is often possible to collect baseline information with brief interventions, whereas there can be difficulties with long-standing or complex programmes where there is no 'blank sheet of paper'. In those cases meaningful background information on the project context can still be collected which will help with the interpretation of results. Ultimately the evaluator needs to decide if baseline information can sensibly be collected and will add substantially to the evaluation.

Monitoring

The requirements for monitoring and its management need to be considered in the planning stages as there is clearly an overlap in terms of setting up systems for monitoring and routinely collecting data for evaluation. Monitoring data can, of course, be collated and used in evaluations. For example, a project might collect details of the age, sex and ethnicity of those registering which could be used to provide evidence about project reach and whether it is accessible to all groups within the community.

↻ **Points for reflection**

Consider a project or programme which you are familiar with. What monitoring data could be easily collected? How could the data be used? What would be the advantages and disadvantages of monitoring?

Monitoring gets little attention in research methods literature yet is an important process which can have positive and negative implications for practice. In an ideal situation, monitoring data would be easily collected, not get in the way of project delivery, and illuminate where there are glitches. In reality many programmes have to cope with burdensome monitoring requirements in order to be accountable to funding bodies. Unless monitoring is considered strategically, there can be a tendency to adopt the maxim 'if it moves, count it' or alternatively abandon monitoring, leaving records incomplete. We suggest that monitoring is considered in developing an evaluation plan so it can be integrated with programme evaluation. In taking a strategic approach, there needs to be consideration of:

• monitoring requirements
• the people involved (both those collecting and volunteering information)
• existing and new data-collection systems
• any potential difficulties and how these could be overcome.

Step 6. Bringing it all together

There is a point in the evaluation where the evidence needs to be brought together. Hopefully, by using an evaluation plan, a lot of relevant evidence will have been gathered and analysed. At this stage, there is a risk that the detail of the findings overwhelms the interpretation. For evaluation to be utilized, key findings need to be identified and the overall strength of the evidence assessed.

In order to judge the success of a programme, the findings should be compared with the original framework of outcomes and indicators. It can be useful to summarize the findings in tabular form, so they can be matched with the indicators. There also needs to be an overview of the project development, implementation and outcomes. Box 4.2 lists a number of key questions which could be asked in an evaluation of a typical small-scale public health project and would serve as a framework for analysis.

The process of interpreting findings can be carried out in conjunction with other stakeholders as it gives people the opportunity to comment on and validate the emerging findings. In their evaluation model, Walden and Baxter (2001) suggest that key strategies include continuous feedback of

> **Box 4.2 Identifying key findings – some questions to consider**
> 1 How has the development of the project been influenced by the context and setting?
> 2 Has the project been delivered as planned?
> 3 Has the project reached its target population?
>   How have stakeholders been involved?
>   Which groups have not been involved?
> 4 Has the project been successful (against its objectives)?
>   What evidence is there? Are there any gaps in evidence?
> 5 Were there any unexpected outcomes?
> 6 What has worked well? Why?
> 7 What has not worked well? Why?
> 8 What lessons have been learnt?
> 9 What aspects would be transferable to other projects?
>   Are there examples of good practice?

findings and seeking a consensus before the final report. Our experience suggests that it is beneficial for practitioners to be involved in this final process of interpretation as it allows some additional reflection to be built into the evaluation and can enable points of learning to emerge.

The final stage of undertaking an evaluation is reporting the findings. Hopefully, by the end of the evaluation, clear and relevant findings will have been identified. Evaluation has a primary purpose to inform practice, and therefore the reporting stage is very significant. Attention to good communication of results will help with utilization of the findings. Chapter 9 discusses some of the challenges of dissemination in more depth. Reporting mechanisms vary with the context of the project, the original purpose of the evaluation and current information needs, but in most instances a written evaluation report will be produced along with other dissemination methods. It can be useful to discuss what type of product is required at the evaluation planning stage. In some ways the report can be seen as the end-point in an evaluation cycle, but equally, as those results are fed back to the project, it could be seen as a starting point for a new cycle of objective setting, data collection and interpretation.

Worked example of an evaluation plan

In Chapter 3 we used the example of a school-based road safety project to speculate on appropriate short-, medium- and long-term outcome indicators through the application of a logical framework. Picking up where we left off, we now show how an evaluation plan can be developed for this project, taking account of steps 1–5 of the framework presented in this chapter. This

time, rather than focusing on educational and behavioural outcomes, we
extend the example to include consideration of environmental and policy
change.

Step 1. Clarifying aims and objectives

The broad aim of the project is to reduce the risk of pedestrian accidents
in children travelling to and from school. Project objectives might
include:

- To enable schools to develop local transport plans in partnership
  with parents, school governors, local residents and other local stakeholders.
- To reduce road hazards in the immediate proximity of participating
  schools.

It is likely that time-frames and targets would be also included – for example,
by 2007, 30 schools will have been recruited to the scheme and developed
transport plans.

Step 2. Choosing indicators

The next stage involves identifying the expected outcomes and indicators.
Table 4.3 shows how an evaluation framework plan would be set out with
different outcome indicators selected.

Step 3. Linking outcomes, indicators, methods

The right-hand column in Table 4.3 identifies how the data will be collected.
Different research methods are shown, but in real life it may be necessary to
agree priorities for data collection.

Step 4. Understanding context and process

Key mechanisms and processes are identified and how these will be measured
(Table 4.4).

Step 5. Setting up data in collection systems

Evaluation planning would involve setting up data-collection systems
and identifying existing data sources. In this example systems to monitor
the adoption of the project within schools and neighbourhoods would be

established. Sources of official road safety statistics would need to be identified, such as accident and emergency attendances. In addition, there may be local consultations and planning surveys which could be accessed.

Step 6. Bringing it all together

At different review points, the evaluator would bring together findings and match these against the indicators of success. It is often helpful to complete the framework with a fifth column so those with an interest in the results can easily see what the criteria for success were, what data were collected and where there is evidence of success. Key findings from the process evaluation and contextual factors can be reported. It is also important that the evaluation captures unanticipated outcomes. In this example the case studies might show that local parents in one area started a successful community campaign to reduce speeding traffic.

Table 4.3 Example of an evaluation framework for a road safety project

Expected outcomes	Activities	Indicators (of success)	How measured?
1. Short term Schools develop transport plans	Partnerships formed Support for planning process	Development of school transport plans	Documentary evidence of transport plans
		Local hazards are identified and plans have agreed actions	Risk assessments completed
		Local policy-makers aware of hazards	Telephone interviews with elected representatives and council officers
2. Medium term Risks removed or minimized near schools	Implementation of agreed actions Meetings with parents and local stakeholders Publication of maps indicating safe routes to school	Changes to environment near schools	Monitoring of agreed changes
		Stakeholders report increased awareness of safe routes to schools	Interviews with stakeholders
		Children and parents able to walk to school using identified safe routes	School survey about travelling to school
		More children walking to school or using public transport	Observation of road use near schools at peak travel periods

Table 4.3 *Cont.*

Expected outcomes	Activities	Indicators (of success)	How measured?
3. Long term Safer local environment for children Reduction of pedestrian accidents	Policy change and maintenance	Fall in number of recorded pedestrian accidents involving children Residents report fewer pedestrian accidents and incidents involving children	Official accident statistics Community mapping of risks, incidents and safe routes

Table 4.4 Example of a process evaluation for a road safety project

What aspects of the process are important?	Questions	How can these be measured?
Motivation to take individual and collective action to improve safety of local environments	How and why did different stakeholders become involved in project? What are the advantages and disadvantages of using safe routes to school?	Semi-structured interviews with key stakeholder groups Focus groups with children and parents
Partnerships with stakeholders	Have strong partnerships been developed? Who is involved? What have been the barriers and facilitating factors?	Interviews with stakeholders Case studies of development of transport plans Records of meetings
Lobbying for policy and environmental change	Has lobbying been successful? Who participated in the campaigns to reduce hazards? What factors influenced local policy change?	Records of meetings Observation of planning progress

Summary

This chapter has presented a framework for planning an evaluation that can be used by those working with small- or medium-scale projects. The framework is intended as a guide to highlight choices and brings a systematic approach to evaluation. Many of the issues raised in this chapter also apply to larger and more complex evaluations. Key points include:

- Evaluation should be planned and carried out in a systematic manner.
- Relevant and appropriate indicators of success should be chosen which will guide the collection of evidence and priorities for data collection.
- It is important to investigate processes and how a project is working.
- Consideration should be given to setting up robust data-collection systems for monitoring and evaluation.

Evaluating community health initiatives

Overview

This chapter provides a guide to evaluating community health initiatives. It covers:

- the nature of community health practice and challenges for evaluation
- guidance on evaluating a community health project
- evaluation of complex community initiatives
- using participatory approaches in evaluation
- suggested resources for undertaking participatory research.

Communities and public health

Community health initiatives have an important place in public health practice. Not only is the community an important setting for health improvement but communities are also seen as a resource for health. Planning and delivering community health programmes creates the need for robust and relevant evaluations. Much of the literature focuses on the challenges of selecting appropriate evaluation methodologies and gathering meaningful evidence of effectiveness. Although we would not wish to underestimate these challenges, evaluating community health initiatives brings rewarding opportunities to research where people live and work and to capture the reality of individual and community change as experienced by different stakeholders. Good evaluation will not only contribute to learning within projects but can be a mechanism to empower communities through building capacity and through the development of shared knowledge (WHO Europe Working Group on Health Promotion Evaluation 1998). This chapter gives a flavour of some of the issues encountered when evaluating community health initiatives and provides guidance on selecting valid and practical approaches, including the use of participatory research methods.

From small community projects to large area programmes, the field of community health reflects diversity in both theory and practice (Tones and Tilford 2001). While some community interventions have a focus on prevention of disease or changing health behaviours, others seek to improve community health and well-being through addressing the wider determinants of health. Banks (2003: 19–20) notes that community practice encompasses five themes:

- equality of opportunity, cultural diversity and social inclusion;
- empowerment of individuals and groups;
- participation;
- partnership and collaborative working;
- mutual learning and growth.

It is these values and concepts that underpin many, but not all, community health initiatives, and this has implications for evaluation.

Point for reflection

How do these values inform the way evaluation is conducted?

Working with communities: some key issues for evaluation

Despite the lack of a unifying model of practice, Fawcett *et al.* (2001: 254–9) identify three major groups of issues for evaluation:

- philosophical or conceptual issues concerning how communities and health problems are defined
- methodological issues concerning the measurement of complexity
- practical, political and ethical issues concerning the conduct and utilization of the evaluation.

Interpreting and defining what is meant by the 'community' in any initiative has theoretical and practical significance (Hawe 1994). Communities can be defined by geographical area or by sharing a common interest or characteristic. At the same time, evaluation has to deal with the diversity within communities, and there may be specific groups that lack visibility. 'Community' can be also used to describe collective action (Butcher 1993) and an evaluation might focus on those community members engaged in shared enterprise rather than the wider community. Overall, evaluators need to be aware of the interpretations of the term 'community' within the context in which they are working, and to have strategies to capture the nature and development of social relations.

Many community health initiatives are based on a holistic model of health, involve multiple partners and have different strands of activity. This presents methodological challenges as the evaluation has to take account of the complexity of practice and be flexible enough to trace developments over time (Potvin and Richard 2001; Rootman *et al.* 2001). Traditional experimentally based methodologies using control groups and randomization are widely regarded as impractical and inappropriate for most community-based initiatives.

Issues concerning community participation and power have implications for evaluation. Firstly, the participation of community members will shape the course of a project as it responds to community needs, and therefore the notion of a standardized intervention is not appropriate. Secondly, the evaluation will need to assess the process of participation as a key mechanism of change. Thirdly, evaluation needs to fit with the values and ethos of the project. The role of the researcher as objective observer and source of expert knowledge, as in the scientific tradition, can be seen to offer a model of research which is disempowering for communities and is clearly at odds with empowering, participatory aims (Hunt 1987; Springett 2001a). In projects where active community participation is a key element, it is recommended that there is also participation in the evaluation (WHO Europe Working Group on Health Promotion Evaluation 1998; Springett 2001a; Hashagen 2003).

In the era of evidence-based practice there is a need for proof of effectiveness. Measuring change in long-term, flexible, community-centred initiatives is challenging. This has sometimes led to tensions between the requirements of funding agencies and those engaged in community health work. Barr (2003) describes the results of extensive consultations with community development practitioners and community representatives. Many reported seeing evaluation as threatening and perceived that external evaluators were failing to understand the complexity of practice and the underlying values. 'As a results of these concerns, many community representatives and front-line workers have felt like victims rather than beneficiaries of evaluation' (Barr 2003: 149). These findings suggest that the need for evidence has to be balanced with an approach to evaluation that is helpful and does not hinder community work.

Evaluating a community health project

Small-scale community health projects are familiar to most public health and health promotion practitioners. Such projects can stand alone but are often part of a wider programme of activities. The challenge is to successfully apply the principles of evaluation in a way which is consistent with the nature of activities and the underlying values. Those involved need to chart a passage through the different stages of evaluation without burdening the project and, at the same time, acknowledge the reality of community practice. Having discussed some of the challenges at the start of this chapter, we now turn our attention to appropriate evaluation approaches for small-scale community projects. Six elements of good practice are identified:

- building evaluation into the project
- maximizing stakeholder involvement
- measuring changes in individual and community health
- using appropriate evaluation methods
- examining processes
- learning in practice.

Building evaluation into the project

There are strong arguments that evaluation in community health projects should be built in from the beginning and undertaken as part of the development process (Baum 1998). While this is recommended for evaluation in general, there are particular advantages here for community health projects as it allows the evaluation to track the development of a project and the way it responds to local needs. Baum (1998) suggests five years as a realistic timeframe, although inevitably many projects will have much shorter life cycles. The integration of evaluation into community practice may lead to different roles for researchers. Beattie (1995) found that evaluations of community development projects were based on approaches which blurred boundaries between the researcher and the researched. In small-scale community projects, evaluation is often done by internal evaluators. However, Kaduskar *et al.* (1999) caution that project workers or volunteers may, quite understandably, lack the confidence and skills to undertake evaluation and therefore training and support should be provided – a point we return to later in this chapter.

Maximizing stakeholder involvement

Those commissioning, managing or undertaking an evaluation of a community health project will need to consider who should be involved and at what stage. The involvement of stakeholders is widely recommended and the range should, as far as is feasible, reflect the type of partnerships in the project. Stakeholders might include community members, representatives from community groups, community workers, local politicians, professionals and managers. Stakeholder involvement can help articulate shared goals and the criteria for success. The Learning Evaluation and Planning (LEAP) framework, for example, involves bringing stakeholders together to agree a 'vision of change for communities' and set locally based indicators (Barr 2003). Judd *et al.* (2001) describe an alternative model where wider stakeholder involvement is used to set standards for community health initiatives which can then be used in evaluations.

Measuring changes in individual and community health

As in any evaluation, indicators of success will be based on project objectives. In many community health projects objectives are very broad at the beginning and become more focused, or indeed change direction, as the project develops. The evaluation should be able to capture changes and identify outcomes from different activities. Both Hunt (1987) and Baum (1998) point out that different stakeholders will have different perspectives on outcomes and these may change over time. An additional challenge is to capture the range of potential outcomes for individuals involved, given the holistic model of health being pursued. For example, in a project developing a community café, some community members may develop confidence and organizational skills and an outcome may be a move to employment. Others involved may report feeling less socially isolated as an outcome. Many projects will be able to give examples of individuals transformed by their involvement, but this may not translate well into the type of evidence required by funding agencies. However, given some creative thinking, it should be possible to devise measurable indicators of success at the individual level.

The measurement of changes in community health and the selection of meaningful community-level indicators is perhaps more challenging. Based on their work with the Canadian Healthy Communities Project, Hayes and Manson Willms (1990: 165) raise concerns that communities are given conflicting messages to 'tackle issues of local concern, but evaluate progress with a common yardstick'. They conclude that one set of indicators is unlikely to fit all projects as the concept of a healthy community will vary from place to place and is dependent on what is valued within communities. While those arguments are cogent, in reality community health projects may lack the capacity to develop tailor-made indicators. Meyrick and Sinkler (1999) provide a set of generic indicators at individual, project and community level which are appropriate for community health projects. An alternative framework is the ABCD (Achieving Better Community Development) model which bases evaluation on the building blocks of community development, leading from aspects of community empowerment to the quality of community life and ultimately the achievement of a healthy, strong community (Barr and Hashagen 2000; Hashagen 2003). Stakeholders are brought together to identify locally relevant indicators within the different dimensions. The strengths of ABCD are that it has been developed with practitioners and offers a comprehensive framework which can be applied flexibly in different contexts.

Using appropriate evaluation methods

The evaluation design and methods have to deal with the complexity and flexibility of community health projects and their interaction with the local environment. We have already noted that experimental designs are generally considered neither appropriate nor feasible. Case study approaches can be used to provide a narrative of the project and the changes that occur in people and the community (Tones and Tilford 2001). Qualitative research methods are favoured as they allow participants to interpret their experiences in their own words, at the same time acknowledging the validity of lay knowledge (Williams and Popay 1994). Community stories have been suggested as a way of reflecting on the developmental processes within communities and understanding changes (Dixon 1995; WHO Regional

Office for Europe 2002), and this approach is discussed further in Chapter 8. There is also the opportunity to use creative methods, such visual arts, as a way of gathering data on projects avoiding reliance on language. Springett (2001a: 146) calls for increased use of observational methods, such as diaries and scrapbooks:

> Extensive and detailed knowledge gained from the systematic observation of the implementation of a programme, in tandem with the tracking of expected effects, can prove useful for the understanding of whether or not and how programmes are effective as health-promotion strategies.

Examining processes

In community health projects, especially those based on community development principles, the processes of participation, capacity building and learning are arguably as important as the outcomes. It is important, therefore, that data are gathered on the quality of those processes during the life of the project. Jewkes (2000) argues that there needs to be a careful examination of the process of participation, looking at who is included and excluded. She suggests that three questions are asked:

- Who participates?
- What is the nature of that participation?
- Whose views prevail?

Other processes that could be examined include:

- the existence of strong networks
- partnerships between services and communities
- development of shared understandings of community health issues
- capacity-building processes
- how social exclusion is addressed.

Learning in practice

Springett (2001a) argues strongly that health promotion evaluation should be about learning and solving practical problems. This has particular pertinence in community health projects where processes facilitate individual and community learning which in turn informs social actions (Springett 2001b). It is therefore appropriate that the evaluation aids learning in projects. Fawcett et al. (2001: 262) contrast two research approaches:

> The traditional evaluation paradigm asks how to configure community conditions, participants and interventions to get an answer to a research question. In contrast, the paradigm of community evaluation asks how to structure the evaluation to understand better and to improve what is important to the community.

Understanding these differing purposes will influence the selection of evaluation strategies for community health projects. Before going on to discuss the evaluation of larger, more complex initiatives, a case study is presented which summarizes the process of evaluation in one project and illustrates some of the challenges involved (see Box 5.1).

Box 5.1 An evaluation of a neighbourhood community health project

The community health project, based in a deprived urban area, had broad aims around redressing inequality, promoting community participation and building intersectoral collaboration. Various community activities were run as part of the project, including a women's group, counselling services, and groups for older people. Members of the local community were involved both as users and as volunteers. The project had been running for a number of years before an evaluation was undertaken.

The evaluation was designed to make a retrospective assessment of what progress the project had made towards the three broad aims. Limited time and resources meant that the evaluation needed to be focused, and a fairly structured approach was taken to gathering evidence on the project activities. In the first instance, a small number of indicators of success were selected, some of them drawn from a generic set of indicators designed for evaluating partnerships (Funnell et al. 1995). The selected indicators acted as a framework to guide data collection with the focus on examining:

• community participation in the project development and current activities
• joint working with other local agencies and organizations
• individual empowerment, looking at the impact on individuals' skills, coping mechanisms and support.

The main research methods were documentary analysis and semi-structured interviews with staff, volunteers and service users. These methods were chosen to generate findings over a short time period and to gain different stakeholder perspectives. Throughout the evaluation, the evaluator worked closely with the project management board and staff. The findings provided a clear assessment of the project and how it was working with individuals and local groups. Points of learning were fed back to the project.

Points for reflection

What were the main challenges faced by the evaluator? Were the main areas of measurement and the data collection methods appropriate for assessing project processes and outcomes? What other areas of measurement could have been included?

Evaluation of complex community initiatives

The principles of community-based evaluation are essentially the same whatever the scale or scope of the programme. Many of the issues raised so far in this chapter apply as much to the evaluation of comprehensive programmes as to small-scale projects. There are, however, additional challenges in evaluating complex community initiatives (see Chapter 3). These could include programmes with a specific focus, such as coronary heart disease prevention, or initiatives addressing the wider social and environmental determinants of health, such as Healthy Cities. In the UK, there has been a plethora of area-based initiatives addressing health and social inequalities, such as Sure Start and New Deal for Communities. This in turn has stimulated interest in the evaluation of complex community initiatives.

Complex community initiatives typically involve different programme strands, multiple partners and a myriad of activities. It is this element of complexity, as opposed to scale or setting, which poses particular problems for evaluation. Health Action Zones can be used to illustrate this point. As we noted in Chapter 3, they were created to tackle health inequalities in areas of deprivation and, like many complex community initiatives, had a strong emphasis on partnership working and community involvement. Typically each HAZ had a mix of activities at programme and project level. In an initial scoping exercise, there were found to be 200 programmes and just under 2000 discrete activities across 26 HAZs (Judge et al. 1999). Barnes et al. (2003) describe the context for evaluation and identify a number of dimensions of complexity within and between HAZs, including: the structures; the range of players; context; blurred boundaries with other work; and the fact that adopted strategies differed between individual programmes/projects and evolved over time.

Much of the debate around evaluation of complex community initiatives focuses on methodological issues. These include:

- the selection of appropriate evaluation approaches to cope with complexity and the open systems of the enterprises (Judge and Bauld 2001)
- the difficulties of randomization (Potvin and Richard 2001)
- the problems of control groups and contamination (Nutbeam et al. 1993)
- measurement of broad social and health outcomes where change might well result after the completion of the initiative (Nutbeam et al. 1993; Mackenzie et al. 2002).

One of the most pertinent problems is attribution and how evaluation can establish a causal link between programme activities and outcomes, given the dynamic environments and the synergy resulting from partnership working (Judge et al. 1999). Henderson et al. (2002: 10), in discussing the evaluation of HAZs, explain how multiple mechanisms impact in multiple contexts resulting in multiple outcomes.

One approach to the evaluation of complex community programmes relies on experimental and quasi-experimental designs, but with attention given to defining the individual components in the programme and understanding how they contribute to the whole (Campbell *et al.* 2000). Hawe *et al.* (2004) argue that what is required is a focus on the function rather than the form in complex interventions. Rather than trying to standardize the individual components of an intervention, what should be standardized is the key steps in the change process, allowing different mechanisms to be selected depending on the context. To use Hawe *et al.*'s example, different research sites would all undertake to develop information tailored to local need, instead of having a standardized health education leaflet. An alternative way of evaluating complex interventions, which has received widespread attention in recent years, is a realist approach based on Theory of Change (Connell and Kubisch 1988) or 'realistic evaluation' (Pawson and Tilley 1997). Theory of Change was indeed developed as an approach for comprehensive community initiatives to overcome the problem of attribution by providing a link between context, purposeful activities and outcomes. The principles of these evaluation approaches are discussed in Section A of this book.

Strategies for local evaluations

Complex community initiatives throw up significant issues for the management and conduct of evaluation in addition to the methodological issues discussed above. In the UK, evaluation (and performance management) requirements for different area-based initiatives have meant that national and local evaluations are undertaken concurrently and data are collected at programme and project level. Figure 5.1 shows an evaluation structure in a typical area-based initiative which illustrates the complexity of assessment and reporting mechanisms. We now highlight some practical strategies for evaluating complex community initiatives at a local level.

Given the complex evaluation structures and the potential range of programme activities, it is important for programmes to adopt a **strategic approach** to the overall evaluation, underpinned by the generic principles of evaluation. Management of competing evaluation demands is needed. There have been reported tensions between national evaluation requirements to assess progress to targets and the need for developmental evaluation to help projects learn (Biott and Cook 2000). Data collection should be planned carefully and priorities selected so that both local and national reporting requirements are met. Mackenzie and Blamey (2005) comment on the potential blurring of roles between the evaluator and programme implementer and also between evaluator and performance manager. This raises the question of what the evaluator's role should be. Should they maintain an objective distance or adopt a supportive – or indeed critically supportive – role? They note the 'formative' responsibility of evaluators to feed back findings which improve programme delivery.

Theory of Change offers a useful framework for evaluation at programme

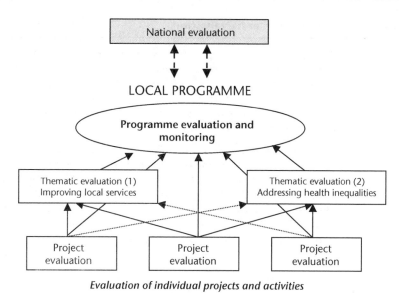

Evaluation of individual projects and activities

Figure 5.1 Evaluation structure in a typical area-based initiative

and project level and has been used extensively in the UK in HAZs and other area-based initiatives. There has been some discussion on the utility of this approach to evaluation. Cotterill (2002) and Bonner (2003) reflect on their experience of supporting evaluation in Plymouth HAZ and identify some of the practical advantages of using Theory of Change as it assists in project planning and also provides a link between the different elements of a programme and the outcomes. Springett and Young (2002), however, point to the time, support and additional facilitation needed to complete a theory of change which may burden small community projects. Good examples of how to develop a theory of change can be found in Hughes and Traynor's (2000) evaluation of a community-based poverty programme and Judge and Bauld's (2001) paper on evaluation of smoking cessation services and capacity for health.

Evaluation capacity is another issue which those with responsibility for evaluation need to consider if project participants, staff and other stakeholders are to become involved in self-evaluation and collecting data on their individual projects. Attention needs to be given to the capacity to undertake evaluation, and additional training and support to projects should be provided (Holden and Downie 2002). This will help ensure that learning from individual projects can inform practice and be fed back into the programme development.

Participatory research and evaluation

Seeking the active engagement of stakeholders in the evaluation process is important for both large- and small-scale community initiatives. There are choices to be made as to the extent of involvement and the adoption of participatory research methods. In this section we highlight some of the advantages and disadvantages of promoting participation in evaluation and examine some practical issues.

'Participatory research' is in effect an umbrella term covering diverse approaches. There is a long tradition of participatory research in health and development (Anyanwu 1988; De Koning and Martin 1996; Rifkin *et al.* 2000), as well as in other contexts such as service evaluations (Boote *et al.* 2002; Beresford 2003) and action research (Hart and Bond 1995; Boutilier *et al.* 1997). Macaulay *et al.* (1999) identify three defining elements of participatory research:

- collaboration
- mutual education
- action (to effect change).

Cornwall and Jewkes (1995) suggest that what really differentiates participatory research from other approaches is the attempt to transfer power from experts to lay people in the research process. While some argue that traditional research approaches, based on objectivity and neutrality, are incongruent with active community engagement (Smithies and Adams 1993), it is possible to incorporate a participatory element within the positivist paradigm, for example in the design and conduct of experimental studies (Hanley *et al.* 2001). Alternatively, emancipatory research strategies, such as participatory action research, promote social action and involve community members in identifying problems, devising, implementing and evaluating solutions (Boutilier *et al.* 1997; Moewaka Barnes 2000; Dickson and Green 2001).

Choosing participatory approaches

The WHO Europe Working Group on Health Promotion Evaluation (1998: 9–10) puts forward some reasons for using participatory approaches:

- They are congruent with the values and principles of health promotion.
- They build people's capacity to address health needs.
- They involve sharing professional and lay resources.
- They encourage a multisectoral approach to the selection of relevant indicators.
- They lead to more relevant and credible evaluation findings and better research utilization.

These arguments are echoed in other literature. Valuing local knowledge and supporting mutual learning are key themes (Feuerstein 1986; Cornwall and Jewkes 1995; Packham 1998). Lay perspectives are likely to differ from professional perspectives and can be incorporated in evaluation (Truman and Raine 2001; Simpson and House 2002). Participatory approaches have particular relevance for evaluation as they engage people in joint action. Furthermore, the findings are more likely to feed into practice because they are grounded in reality (Springett 2001b). As we discuss in Chapter 7, participatory research can offer a mechanism to access marginalized and disadvantaged communities without reinforcing inequalities (Moewaka Barnes 2000; Brodie 2003).

There are disadvantages to using participatory approaches in evaluation. Allison and Rootman (1996) discuss one of the most fundamental challenges – that of achieving rigour when the researcher does not have full control of the research process. Participatory approaches are not recommended where an evaluation is very complex or involves methods requiring technical expertise (Krueger and King 1998). Demands for certain types of evidence may mean it is more important for communities to be involved in identifying research priorities rather than in the conduct of evaluation. The thorny issue of representativeness is put forward as another disadvantage, as those actively engaged will be atypical and this may impact on the validity of the evaluation (Entwistle *et al.* 1998; Boote *et al.* 2002). As well as methodological challenges, there are practical limitations which may influence the adoption of participatory approaches. Participatory methods are time-consuming and resource-intensive, and community capacity to undertake evaluation may be limited. Nguyet Nguyen and Otis (2003) describe the experience of attempting to increase citizen participation in a large-scale evaluation of a heart health programme. They encountered a number of problems, including: patchy involvement leading to gaps in data; lack of community interest in evaluation; community volunteers feeling overwhelmed; inadequate time and budget to build trust; and conflicts with evaluation requirements.

↻ Points for reflection

Holman (1987) and Tandon (1996) both assert that research is not a politically neutral process.

Whose interests are being served by undertaking an evaluation?

Who participates in an evaluation and why?

What can be done to address the power imbalances between professionals and lay people in evaluation?

Where the active engagement of community members or service users is sought in evaluation, there must be clarity of purpose and transparency about the level of power sharing involved. There is a great deal of rhetoric

about community participation in research, but full community control of
an evaluation may be neither achievable nor desirable. Krieger *et al.* (2002)
suggest that there is a spectrum of methods which should be selected according to the individual project, taking into account the potential community
benefits and the need to promote good-quality research and facilitate stakeholder involvement. We have applied Wilcox's (1994) ladder of participation
to evaluation activities to illustrate different levels of participation in the
evaluation process (Table 5.1). Cornwall and Jewkes (1995) make the point
that levels of participation may fluctuate at different points in a research
project.

Table 5.1 Levels of participation in evaluation

	Level 1	Level 2	Level 3	Level 4	Level 5
	Information giving	Consultation	Decision making	Acting together	Supporting community initiatives
Typical process	Presentation and promotion	Communication and feedback	Consensus building	Partnership building	Capacity building
Evaluation activities – examples	Attending community meetings and events to explain the evaluation and answer questions	Consulting over questionnaire design to check questions are relevant and appropriate	Community representatives on a project board deciding evaluation priorities for a project	Community members working alongside professionals to undertake data collection	Offering training and support to community groups to help them self-evaluate
	Producing clear information which is accessible to all	Setting up a reference group to advise on aspects of the evaluation	Different stakeholders working together to select indicators of success	Planning and working together on a dissemination event	Integrating research with community development

Some practical issues

Using participatory approaches in evaluation requires forethought. What
can be an exciting and ultimately rewarding experience has the potential to
go badly wrong and may affect trust between different stakeholders. Some of
the practical issues that need consideration before embarking on participatory evaluation are as follows:

- *Training.* Participation in evaluation will normally require some training
  or educational element to prepare people for evaluation activities and to
  develop research skills. Training may focus solely on technical issues, but
  Meulenberg-Buskens (1996) recommends that it is seen as an integral part

of the process of shared learning and involves developing skills in critical reflection.

- *Skills of the evaluation team*. Professionals and researchers involved in carrying out a participatory evaluation will require good facilitation skills and be comfortable with a flexible, people-centred approach to research (Anyanwu 1988). Brodie (2003) suggests that those commissioning evaluation will want to ensure that evaluation teams have the relevant experience in community research. Evaluators will also require good group skills.
- *Recruitment*. There can be problems in recruiting and retaining local people to act as community researchers (Parry *et al.* 2001; Lever and Moore 2004). Therefore strategies to overcome these potential difficulties need to be in place. There are decisions about whether community researchers remain as volunteers or are employed. While clearly people should be recompensed for their efforts, the whole question of payment for community research is a very difficult one, complicated by the benefits system in the UK (Brodie 2003; INVOLVE 2003).
- *Documenting the process*. Participatory approaches require attention to the process as well as the outcomes of research and often involve the use of collective methods such as community mapping or art works. It is important that there is good documentation as the project progresses (Tolley and Bentley 1996).
- *Offering support*. Time is needed to build relationships and trust (Sullivan *et al.* 2001), and also to develop cohesive, functioning collaborations. People new to the world of evaluation need to develop confidence and understanding in order to make a contribution. Adequate time and resources should be allocated to support participatory evaluation. This will help ensure that evaluation capacity is built within the community rather than the expertise staying 'locked up' and the community remaining dependent on external evaluators for future evaluations (Feuerstein 1986: 12).

Further information on using participatory approaches can be found in the resources suggested in Box 5.2. Cornwall and Jewkes (1995: 1668) highlight the 'personal, political and professional challenges' raised by the practice of participatory research. While few would suggest it is an easy option for evaluation, the potential benefits should be considered. Writing about their research with Aboriginal grandmothers, Dickson and Green (2001: 481) explain: 'when provided with the opportunity, tools, and support, ordinary people can indeed conduct research that is meaningful to them and contributes to personal and social change'.

Box 5.2 Resources for participatory evaluation

INVOLVE aims 'to promote and support active public involvement in NHS, public health and social care research'. The group's web pages [www.invo.org.uk].give access to a range of publications that offer clear, practical guidance on participation in research: these include:

Getting involved in research – a guide for consumers (Royle et al. 2001)

Involving the public in NHS, public health, and social care research: briefing notes for researchers (Hanley et al. 2004)

A guide to paying members of the public actively involved in research (INVOLVE 2003).

Other useful resources include:

Partners in evaluation. Evaluating development and community programmes with participants (Feuerstein 1986)

The involvement of parents and carers in Sure Start local evaluations (Brodie 2003)

Participatory approaches in health promotion and health planning. A literature review (Rifkin 2000)

Summary

Working with communities to improve health is part and parcel of public health practice. This chapter has considered some of the methodological and practical issues around collecting evidence in the community setting. Key points include the following:

- Evaluation can help build capacity in community projects and aid learning.
- Measurement of changes should be based on a holistic model of health and indicators selected at individual and community level.
- Complex community initiatives require a strategic approach to evaluation.
- Where projects are using community development approaches, appropriate research methods should be used to gather evidence.
- Involving lay people in evaluation can bring benefits, but training and support may need to be offered.

6 Ethics and evaluation

Overview

This chapter identifies key ethical considerations for public health and health promotion evaluation. It includes:

- principles guiding ethical practice in evaluation
- ethical issues encountered in the commissioning, design, conduct and dissemination of evaluation
- research governance and ethics in the NHS
- roles and responsibilities in research partnerships.

Research, ethics and evaluation

Research ethics is concerned with the relationship between the researcher and the researched and the moral principles underpinning research actions. Research and evaluation are not neutral processes but take place in social contexts where ethical dilemmas inevitably arise. Those engaged in evaluation should be willing to go to lengths to protect individuals' rights and be sensitive to potential abuses of power. In the UK, the emergence of various health scandals and increasing public mistrust of 'science' has resulted in heightened awareness of ethical issues and changes in the governance of health research (Beresford 2003). Undoubtedly evaluation practice is subject to greater scrutiny than ever before.

Evaluation involves research activity and therefore research ethics needs to be considered at all stages of the evaluation process: in commissioning, managing and conducting evaluation and in the way the results are reported, disseminated and utilized. Kent (2000a) describes the four ethical principles which govern research practice:

- **autonomy** – individuals' rights to self-determination should be respected;
- **beneficence** – the research should contribute to the public good;
- **non-maleficence** – the research should not result in any harm (physical, social or psychological);
- **justice** – the research itself and the treatment of those involved should be fair and equitable.

Drawing on a human rights approach (LoBiondo-Wood and Haber 1994), Eby (2000) identifies how research should protect human rights to self-determination, to privacy and dignity, to anonymity and confidentiality, to fair treatment and to protection from discomfort and harm. Human rights and the four ethical principles form the basis for international and national codes of research ethics. The most relevant ones for public health and health promotion are the Helsinki Declaration for biomedical research (World Medical Association 2004) and the ethical guidelines of the Social Research Association (2003) and the British Psychological Society (2004).

All those engaged in evaluation need to have a basic understanding of research ethics, and there is an extensive literature in this field. Ethical principles are enshrined in some of the norms of research practice: the need for informed consent, protecting the anonymity of research participants, ensuring results are reported truthfully and so on. Whilst established practice can provide guidance to those involved in evaluation, there are always cases where ethical dilemmas arise, either where principles are in conflict or where there are questions about how best to put principles into operation. Kent (2000a: 62) suggests that ethics and moral theory cannot tell a researcher what to do faced with specific circumstances:

> Although ethics helps the researcher to understand better this ethically problematic situation, it only provides a framework for making decisions. Ultimately the researcher has to draw upon his or her values and experiences and the cultural context when considering what action to take in response to an ethical dilemma.

Gallagher *et al.* (1995) highlight how solutions to ethical dilemmas can in turn raise methodological and practical issues. They discuss the merits of taking a pragmatic approach to ethical conflicts whereby judgements are based on an assessment of the relative significance of different ethical principles within the actual research setting.

Ethics in evaluation practice

Evaluation is a research activity and at the same time part of professional practice. The nature of public health and health promotion raises some unique ethical issues. Indeed, Elliston (2002) suggests that health promotion research, because of its multidisciplinary nature, requires a tailored code of ethics. The ethics of professional practice undoubtedly influence the conduct of evaluation in practice settings. In this section we identify some of the major ethical issues for evaluation and pose four key questions relating to different stages of the evaluation process. There is also a case study, drawn from public health practice, which illustrates some real life dilemmas (Box 6.1).

↻ **Points for reflection**

What key values guide your interactions with people in your work setting?

What implications does that have for the way evaluation should be approached?

Question 1: Commissioning evaluation – is it ethical to evaluate?

The fundamental question of whether an evaluation should be undertaken can itself raise ethical dilemmas. As we indicated in Chapter 1, there are a number of justifications for evaluation, but there may also be reasons why it is unethical to proceed. Reasons include where:

- evaluation would not represent an ethical use of resources because it would divert time, staff and funds from essential activities;
- evaluation would place an unacceptable burden on practitioners and other stakeholders;
- communities or organizations have been over-researched and do not want to be evaluated;
- evaluation would be too intrusive or risk generating conflict in areas of work where there are major social, political or cultural tensions;
- it is not possible to carry out an evaluation of sufficient depth and quality to aid decision-making;
- evaluators would be compromised and would not be free to report findings accurately.

Alternatively, there are strong moral grounds for arguing that all public health and health promotion activity should be evidence-based. A key question is whether it is ethical to continue to carry out initiatives without evaluating if they are acceptable, reach the right people, are effective and do no harm. However, Wright (1999) makes the point that there are cases where it is better not to do an evaluation at all if only poor quality evidence will be produced or the results will be ignored. Sometimes there are ethical dilemmas between the need for knowledge to benefit wider society, informed by utilitarian principles, and considering the impact for those directly involved in local projects. For example, a head teacher and school governors would be dealing with an ethical dilemma in deciding whether a school should act as a pilot for a drugs prevention package. Evaluation of the pilot would provide evidence which others could use but may not directly benefit pupils or the school. Overall, the need for evidence has to be balanced with consideration of wider moral issues and whether appropriate safeguards can be put in place to protect participants.

Question 2: Are experimental designs ethical in public health and health promotion?

The need to generate evidence in order to underpin ethical professional practice has led some evaluators to select experimental designs for evaluation. Putting aside the methodological and practical issues discussed earlier in the book, experiments raise specific ethical issues because the research designs are based on control, manipulation and randomization, and the intervention is normally withheld from some groups (Stephenson and Imrie 1998). Randomization and blinding, seen as important to ensure internal validity, raise ethical issues in terms of informed consent and rights to self-determination (Davies *et al.* 2000; Oakley *et al.* 2003). The ethics of randomized controlled trials rests on what is termed 'collective equipoise', where there is collective (and genuine) uncertainty about which intervention is best and consent is obtained on that basis (Edwards *et al.* 1998). While RCTs have an assured place in public health research, it is fair to say that there are sharp divisions of opinion about the ethics of using them within health promotion (see WHO Europe Working Group on Health Promotion Evaluation 1998; Oakley 1998b; Oakley *et al.* 2003). Alternative designs which raise fewer ethical problems can be selected, such as natural experiments, where there is comparison between areas that happen to be using different approaches (St Leger *et al.* 1992: 108–9).

Question 3: Conducting the evaluation – how can participants be protected?

Whatever design or methods are chosen, evaluations should be conducted ethically and within the relevant legal framework. As a minimum, attention should be given to aspects such as consent procedures, ensuring people have adequate information and protecting anonymity. Ultimately the evaluation needs to be based on trust between the various actors. It is important ethically that the evaluation does not interfere with or undermine activities and relationships within initiatives. Oliver (2003: 84–6) argues that those engaged in any research should try to maintain what he terms the 'social ecology' of a setting.

Public health and health promotion programmes are routinely working with people who have reduced access to health resources or who are marginalized, and this can raise additional ethical issues. Without care it is easy for professionals and researchers to exert power through the evaluation process. The conduct of the evaluation should ensure that inequalities are not exacerbated and that people are not made to feel disempowered. Sensitive topics may vary with social contexts and will need to be dealt with accordingly (Lee 1993). Using participatory approaches can throw open a number of ethical issues. Minkler (2004) argues that community-based participatory research in public health is consistent with values of social justice and self-determination, but identifies ethical challenges at various stages of the research process. These challenges include:

- achieving a genuine community-driven agenda
- dealing with inside–outsider tensions
- the limitations of who participates
- 'cultural misunderstandings' and the impact of racism in communities
- issues around ownership and dissemination of findings when faced with resistance from the community.

While Minkler highlights these issues for participatory approaches, the more general point is that evaluators should not breeze in and out of projects with little regard for participants' needs and aspirations.

Question 4: How are results disseminated and used?

Ethical issues can surface at the dissemination phase, and Øvretveit (1998: 198) discusses how evaluators have a duty to report findings and ensure results are not misinterpreted. Publication of results from an evaluation may have benefits in terms of learning and increased visibility for projects, but it can also have unwanted consequences where negative results are reported or tensions are present. Holman (1987) argues that research is an instrument of power affecting the distribution of resources. Evaluations are used to make decisions on funding, and that can mean that those evaluating a project may find themselves caught between the agendas of different stakeholders. Whitehead (1993) raises questions about who really owns the research (the funders, the researchers, the community or the wider public) and how they control the dissemination process. There are perhaps no easy answers to these dilemmas except to ensure some transparency about the purpose of the evaluation and how information will be used. The challenges for dissemination are discussed further in Chapter 9.

Box 6.1 Evaluation of a health bus for young people (Salvin 2004)

The evaluation concerned an outreach service offering health advice to young people aged 13–19 years. The aims of the service were to reduce teenage pregnancy and to provide information on issues of concern to young people in a safe, confidential and welcoming environment. Monitoring data indicated that the health bus was well used, particularly by young males. As the initiative had been running for a few years, it was felt important to evaluate the service in order to inform decisions about future funding. The practitioner with responsibility for the evaluation, who also had a role in managing the initiative, wanted to focus the evaluation on obtaining the views of young males, as traditionally members of that group are reluctant to access services. A qualitative approach using individual interviews was chosen to allow the young men to talk about their experiences. One major difficulty for the evaluation was that the service on the bus was completely confidential and no records of contact details were kept.

Approval to undertake the evaluation was obtained from the local NHS Research Ethics Committee. The practitioner conducting the evaluation faced a number of ethical dilemmas, and the following are some of the strategies adopted to address these:

- Recruitment was carried out through flyers advertising 'drop-in' research sessions on particular days.
- Participants were self-nominated but a small incentive was offered.
- Interviews were conducted in a private, soundproof area on the bus.
- Confidentiality was assured in line with the service guidelines, but this meant parents were not approached for consent.
- The interview schedule was carefully developed to avoid disclosure of personal information.

Extremely useful, and to some extent unexpected, findings emerged from the evaluation. It had been assumed that the setting was the reason behind the success in attracting young men, but in fact the results indicated that it was the service approach which was more important. These findings enabled decisions to be made about use of resources, and the provision offered by the bus was expanded to include new areas of need.

Points for reflection

What were the ethical issues at the different stages of the evaluation?

Were there tensions between ethical, methodological and practical concerns? How could these be resolved?

Did this evaluation adhere to ethical principles? Consider alternative approaches.

Some common themes

In examining the ethics of evaluation and the issues raised by the case study in Box 6.1, three underlying themes emerge:

- the push for evidence
- evaluation embedded in practice
- a focus on health inequalities.

The first theme relates to the context in which evidence is produced and the ethical tensions resulting from the drive for evidence-based practice. Questions are thrown up around the ethics of small-scale evaluations, the selection of methodologies, the type of evidence demanded and created, and how it is used in making decisions about the allocation of resources. These issues have relevance in any evaluation research but have particular resonance in the fields of public health and health promotion which carry a 'burden of proof' to justify activity.

The second theme concerns the ethics of evaluation in professional practice. Evaluation is often differentiated from research on the basis that evaluation is primarily about local knowledge for action. However, in professional practice it may be hard to draw the boundary between research and evaluation, and this can affect what code of practice people operate by. The fact that evaluation is integral to practice does not absolve practitioners from considering research ethics, indeed some participatory approaches common in practice raise ethical issues not encountered in traditional research. In addition, partnership working may present ethical issues for evaluation as different stakeholders approach ethical dilemmas in different ways and those with responsibility for evaluation may not have complete control over the conduct of the research.

Finally, the concern to address health inequalities has implications for evaluation practice. Charting an ethical path in some of the contexts for practice can be daunting. The case study in Box 6.1 illustrates some of the challenges of evaluating an outreach service. The practitioner involved had a choice to engage with those issues or not evaluate. Faced a similar dilemma in their evaluation of a counselling service for children and young people, Horrocks and Blyth (2003: 22) concluded: 'the worst possible outcome would have been to deny the young people the opportunity to have their views listened to and have such views incorporated into improving services'. Ultimately, ethics in practice means that evaluation has to reflect and not undermine core values of health promotion and public health.

Research governance and ethical review

In the UK all health research is undertaken within a legal framework and may be subject to NHS ethical review. Similar review systems exist in other countries and are designed primarily to protect the public. The NHS Research Governance framework (Department of Health 2001a: 3) states: 'The public has a right to expect high scientific, ethical and financial standards, transparent decision-making processes, clear allocation of responsibilities and robust monitoring arrangements'. Those engaged in evaluation need to be aware of the systems designed to safeguard people and the standards that are expected within the public domain. Box 6.2 summarizes ethical review in the NHS. The wider legal framework on issues such as confidentiality and intellectual property rights should be also heeded (Townend 2000). The **Data Protection Act 1998** is particularly relevant as it covers the processing and storage of personal data in both electronic and manual records, and that includes data obtained for monitoring and evaluation purposes. Obligations placed on those handling data include ensuring such data are accurate, relevant, not excessive and stored securely (Information Commissioner n.d.). Information on the Act can be found at http://www.informationcommissioner.gov.uk/. Boyd (2003) and Myers *et al.* (2004) discuss some of the practical implications of accessing and using health information in research.

Box 6.2 Ethical review in the NHS

The **Research Governance Framework** (Department of Health 2005b) sets standards for the conduct of health research to improve the quality of research and to prevent poor practice, misconduct and fraud. It covers five domains:

- ethics
- science
- information on research (including dissemination)
- health, safety and employment
- finance and intellectual property.

Research and development approval through local NHS trusts is required for any research, clinical or non-clinical, taking place in the NHS or involving NHS patients or staff. Further information is available from http://www.dh.gov.uk/ PolicyAndGuidance/ResearchAndDevelopment/ResearchAndDevelopmentAZ/ ResearchGovernance/fs/en.

A network of **research ethics committees** (RECs), overseen by the Central Office for Research Ethics Committees (COREC), exists to review research. The RECs are independent committees with a mix of lay, professional and academic members who meet regularly to review research proposals to ensure that they meet ethical principles and are scientifically sound (Central Office for Research Ethics Committees n.d.). Researchers submit a form describing how they will deal with ethical issues and giving full details on aspects such as research methods, recruitment, consent and data protection. Extensive guidance on the process can be found at: http://corec.org.uk

---

Ethical approval for evaluation

Few would argue with the view that all evaluation should be professionally conducted to acceptable quality standards and should adhere to ethical principles. However, there are questions about the applicability of research governance arrangements to evaluation. Ethical review can present unnecessary bureaucratic hurdles for small-scale evaluation and be very time-consuming. Some have argued that review processes in the NHS, geared to assess biomedical research, are not suited to the review of qualitative research (Tod *et al.* 2002) or low-risk, community-based social research (MacPherson *et al.* 2005). On the other hand, review provides scrutiny and can prevent abuses taking place. Thurston *et al.* (2003) suggest that ethical review offers a mechanism of accountability and there should be review when evaluation is judging the effectiveness of an intervention, as opposed to evaluation as quality assurance where the aim is to assess the implementation of an intervention known to be effective.

In the NHS, research is defined as 'the attempt to derive generalisable new knowledge by addressing clearly defined questions with systematic and rigorous methods' (Department of Health 2005b: 3). Not all the evaluation undertaken within public health practice would fall within that definition, but evaluators will need to seek local advice. Demonstration projects where evidence will be disseminated nationally will undoubtedly require ethical approval. On the other hand, small-scale evaluations undertaken with the purpose of checking that projects are going to plan and informing local action can be classed as service evaluation and as such do not require ethical review under the current arrangements (NHS Research and Development Forum 2005). Table 6.1 shows how research and service evaluation are differentiated for the purposes of deciding if a project requires formal NHS ethical review. Although the typology is framed in terms of clinical research and practice, the classification could be extended to public health and health promotion. Where the evaluation is dealing with sensitive issues or involves vulnerable people, such as children, then it is safe to assume that ethical review will be required. There are further complications for public health evaluation, as partnership working can mean stakeholders relate to different organizational boundaries and systems. Those with responsibility for evaluation, who are faced with negotiating different processes to gain approval, may choose to consult with local managers to assess the position in their area.

Table 6.1 Differences between research and evaluation

Research	Service evaluation
Motivated to generate new knowledge	Motivated to define current care
Quantitative research is hypothesis-based Qualitative research explores themes using established methodology	Designed to answer the question 'what standard does this service achieve?'
May involve a new treatment	Does not involve a new treatment
May involve additional therapies, samples and investigations	Involves no more than administration of interview, questionnaires or record analysis
May involve allocation to treatment groups	Does not involve allocation to treatment groups: the health professional or patient chooses
May involve randomization	Does not involve randomization

Source: http://www.corec.org.uk

Consent procedures in evaluation

One area where differences exist in practice is that of informed consent. Informed consent is a cornerstone of research ethics and involves the researcher in:

- providing clear and sufficient information about the research
- checking potential participants understand what is involved and are competent to consent
- obtaining voluntary consent (Kent 2000b).

Consent procedures for research tend to be quite formal, usually requiring written consent, but may be more relaxed for evaluation in professional practice (Celnick 2000). For example, participants in a training programme may take part in a focus group as an integral part of that programme and may not be asked to consent separately as they would for a research project. Similar issues arise with action research, where there can be a lack of clarity over whether people are consenting to the change or the research (Eby 2000). Consent procedures can have real practical and ethical implications for evaluation. MacQueen and Buehler (2004) describe the evaluation of an initiative to improve HIV prevention services where some departments sought ethical approval and put in place formal consent procedures suitable for clinical research. They suggest that such procedures were too complex and caused unnecessary distress and confusion given the low risk to service users. Evaluators have to be prepared to adapt the principles of informed consent to the specific context while being sensitive to the needs of participants. Giving good information (see Box 6.3) and respecting autonomy do not necessarily mean imposing formal consent procedures. Written consent may be particularly problematic for some groups, such as those with low literacy or with a fear of bureaucracy (for example asylum seekers). Insistence on written consent may result in excluding some groups from taking part in evaluation, which is in itself questionable on ethical grounds.

Further issues arise with population- or community-level interventions where there are questions of who is classed as a participant and how consent can be obtained. Where clusters (such as schools) are used for sampling, initial consent is given by gatekeepers acting in the interests of the population, although there is increasing emphasis on obtaining individual consent for data collection at a later stage. Edwards *et al.* (1999) argue that there should be procedural safeguards for sampling clusters, and guardians should only volunteer groups or populations when issues of justice, utility and equity have been considered.

Box 6.3 What should be included on a consent form

- The purpose of the evaluation
- Information about the people and organization doing the evaluation
- Information that participation is voluntary
- What information will be requested
- Whether there is any risk to participants
- How the information will be gathered
- Who will have access to the information
- How confidentiality will be assured
- How the information will be used
- Contact details

Source: Health Communication Unit 2006: 49

Standards for evaluation

As we noted in Chapter 1, evaluation undertaken within public health practice is not the same as conducting an academic research study, although a minority of projects will serve both purposes. While ethical review systems may provide some scrutiny, many evaluations will not go through those procedures. In these cases other governance mechanisms should ensure accountability to the immediate stakeholders, including those commissioning the evaluation, and to a lesser extent to the public, professional and research communities. Where approval is sought from external organizations, the evaluator should identify appropriate individuals with the authority to make the necessary decisions on the evaluation.

There are strong arguments for developing quality standards for good evaluation practice. National standards exist such as those produced by the Canadian Evaluation Society (n.d.). The UK Evaluation Society (2003b) includes guidelines for self-evaluation as well as for those commissioning evaluation. Alternatively, standards could be developed within local organizations. The American Evaluation Association (2004) has five succinct guiding principles for evaluators:

1 *Systematic inquiry.* Evaluators conduct systematic, data-based inquiries about whatever is being evaluated.
2 *Competence.* Evaluators provide competent performance to stakeholders.
3 *Integrity/honesty.* Evaluators ensure the honesty and integrity of the entire evaluation process.
4 *Respect for people.* Evaluators respect the security, dignity and self-worth of the respondents, programme participants, clients, and other stakeholders.
5 *Responsibilities for general and public welfare.* Evaluators articulate and take into account the diversity of interests and values that may be related to the general and public welfare.

Collaborative evaluation – roles and responsibilities

Practitioners' roles and responsibilities in evaluation can vary. South and Tilford's (2000) three models of research in practice can be applied to evaluation:

- *integration*, where practitioners undertake small-scale evaluation as part of routine practice;
- *consumers*, where practitioners draw on existing evidence and may commission evaluation;
- *partnership*, where practitioners are engaged in dialogue with researchers, collaborate on evaluation activities and act in a consultative capacity on projects.

The integration and consumer models can be seen to fit with choices over whether evaluation is conducted by internal or external evaluators who would then have the primary responsibility for ensuring that ethical and quality issues are addressed. Internal evaluators may of course find themselves caught between professional and research obligations (Crow 2000). In the case of the partnership model, roles and responsibilities for evaluation may be less clear-cut, and this can have ethical, methodological and political implications. It is this aspect we consider now.

Collaborative evaluation as a term encompasses various types of evaluation, including participatory evaluation approaches and action research as well as collaborations which have less direct involvement in the planning and conduct of the evaluation. Ross *et al.* (2003) identify three levels for the involvement of decision-makers in research:

- as formal supporters
- as a responsive audience giving suggestions and information
- as an integral partner with active involvement in aspects of the research process.

There are sound reasons for adopting collaborative models in evaluation, as we identified in Chapter 5. It is argued that partnerships in research are more likely to result in relevant research with findings used directly in policy and practice (Walter *et al.* 2003). Pollitt (1999), however, raises a number of concerns about collaborative evaluation. He argues that the rejection of an independent, expert stance in favour of a pluralistic approach to evaluation may compromise the rigour of the research. Achieving a consensus in evaluation may not be possible or it may reduce the impact of the findings: 'Sharp corners and uncomfortable comparison may be drafted out in the interests of consensualism. Vagueness and fudge sometimes turn out to be the common denominators' (Pollitt 1999: 86). Finally, he identifies ethical tensions which may arise in trying to represent all views and the possibility of conflicts between interests of major stakeholders and the public good.

Even where collaborative evaluation is underpinned by a strong rationale and there are clear, identified benefits, there can be risks for those involved.

One example drawn from our experience illustrates some of these issues. The evaluation focused on the work of a small district team working in local health organizations (South and Green 2001). A collaborative approach was taken, with some shared data collection and regular meetings between the external evaluators and the team. Findings were used directly to shape the development of the work and were fed into different local forums. There were, however, considerable and conflicting responsibilities placed on all involved. The team members had a responsibility to report their experiences 'warts and all' to enable learning to occur, but they could not easily hide behind a cloak of anonymity in their respective organizations. The evaluators had responsibilities to report accurately and feed results back to the various forums and organizations without exposing individuals. There were risks that the close collaboration could have undermined the validity of the evaluation or the work of the team. It was essential to build a relationship of trust, with opportunities for open and honest dialogue. In addition, a clear ethical statement about access to data, confidentiality and feedback of findings was agreed with team members and was used to guide the conduct of the evaluation.

Overall, collaborative evaluation may be a natural choice for public health and offer undoubted benefits, but the ethical implications need to be taken into account. Risks should be identified and managed appropriately. It is important that responsibilities are negotiated between the different partners, and aspects such as management and conduct of the evaluation, quality standards and dissemination are addressed.

Summary

Ethics needs to be considered at all stages of evaluation from commissioning to dissemination. While practice should be guided by ethical principles and respect for human rights, this chapter has shown that ethical issues in evaluation are rarely simple and few clear-cut solutions exist. Those engaged in public health evaluation need to be aware of the debates and be prepared to address ethical concerns. The chapter has highlighted a number of issues, including:

• tensions around the push for evidence and responsibilities for ensuring good-quality evaluation
• the need to protect vulnerable groups and allow them the opportunity to participate in evaluation
• managing informed consent within practice
• ethical review and research governance frameworks
• roles and responsibilities in collaborative evaluation.

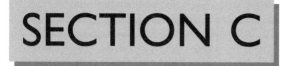

SECTION C

Challenges

7 | Evaluation with hard-to-reach groups

Overview

This chapter considers evaluation with hard-to-reach groups. It includes:

- identifying hard-to-reach groups
- real-life dilemmas and case studies from practice
- practical research strategies for involving hard-to-reach groups
- evaluating access and reach
- the power of evaluation.

Hidden problems and excluded groups

Public health endeavour is not simply directed to health improvement but involves addressing health inequalities and promoting equity. Work to engage and support the more marginalized groups in society throws up major challenges for evaluation practice. In this chapter we consider some of the most significant issues and identify useful strategies. Before addressing some of the practicalities and dilemmas, we need to ask what is meant by a 'hard-to-reach group'? Evidently any group of people can be hard to reach, depending on the specific context. Busy clinical staff, for example, may be difficult to engage in a health promotion initiative. More often the term 'hard-to-reach' is used to describe individuals and communities who are marginalized and not able to fully benefit from mainstream services. People facing barriers to maintaining and improving their health include identifiable groups, such as asylum seekers, and groups which lack visibility because of stigma or hidden needs. Thinking more widely, there are many individuals who may be targeted by a public health initiative but are simply unaware or choose not to participate. Social exclusion is used as 'a shorthand term for what can happen when people or areas suffer from a combination of linked problems such as unemployment, poor skills, low incomes, poor housing, high crime, bad health and family breakdown', the key characteristic being the way problems are 'mutually reinforcing' (Social Exclusion Unit 2001: 10).

↻ Points for reflection

Consider a familiar area of public health. Identify who is hard-to-reach in that context and why. What challenges does that pose for research?

Hard-to-reach groups pose two major challenges for evaluation in practice. The first challenge concerns assessing effectiveness, especially where programmes aim to include marginalized groups. Evaluation has a role is assessing whether programmes have reached their target population, are accessible and inclusive, address needs adequately, and are making a contribution to tackling health inequalities. Given the values of public health and health promotion, these questions need to be addressed, but they are not always easy to answer well. Later in the chapter, we consider how access and reach can be measured.

The second challenge concerns the conduct of evaluation in real-life situations. If some groups are hard to reach or not known to services, then, in most cases, they are also hard to reach for the purposes of research. Genuine barriers may exist which will constrain or even prevent evaluation from taking place. Differences in language, culture, abilities, age, and so on, may present practical difficulties and undermine the process of collecting valid data. Where strategies are not put in place, the risk is that evaluation will result in some voices being ignored. As we have argued earlier, it is critical that evaluation does not undermine public health practice and exacerbate inequalities. We now examine three dilemmas, drawn from real-life projects, which are used to illustrate some of the problems commonly encountered. For each dilemma, the actual solution which was adopted is described and emerging issues highlighted.

Common dilemmas for evaluation

Dilemma 1: Dealing with diversity

Dilemma 1 concerns a community survey of parents which assessed satisfaction with local services and was undertaken as part of the evaluation of a Sure Start local programme (Newell *et al.* 2004). The Sure Start area was ethnically diverse; the Census indicated that 30 per cent of the population were from ethnic minorities. Many families were new to the area and these included asylum seekers, international students and people not known to the statutory authorities. In one of the local primary schools, 22 languages were spoken. The evaluators needed to ensure that the survey was broadly representative and people were not excluded from taking part because of language or cultural barriers, but on the other hand, there were limited resources available. Translation of the questionnaires was not considered a practical option due to the range of languages spoken, and there was patchy access to interpreting services. Furthermore, it was predicted that literacy would be a problem across all sections of the community. Other issues were the desire to obtain the views of parents not registered with the programme and the absence of a list of all families living in the area which could have acted as a sample frame (a complete list of potential participants from which a sample is drawn). These types of issues concerning diversity, language barriers and hidden communities are commonly faced by programmes and have implications for evaluation. The solution adopted here was to train a group of parents to administer the questionnaire in places where parents were meeting and also in their immediate neighbourhoods. In addition, community outreach workers employed by the Sure Start programme, including a Chinese link worker, went knocking on doors. It was felt that having a local parent or community worker administering the questionnaire would help bypass literacy barriers. Overall the approaches adopted were very labour-intensive and therefore the coverage was both limited and also skewed to areas where people had existing contacts. The strategy of involving local parents was successful at finding families not registered with the programme, but the restricted range of languages spoken by the volunteers was reflected in the coverage of the survey. Although the ethnic breakdown of respondents broadly matched the Census figures, results indicated that there was only partial success at reaching people where language barriers existed.

⟳ Points for reflection

What were the strengths and limitations of using the strategies adopted above?

What additional methods could have been used which might have overcome language barriers?

Should community surveys be attempted if it is not possible to reach all sections of the target population?

Projects that work exclusively with specific ethnic groups will often have access to experienced interpreters, but such specialist resources are not always available when evaluating programmes working across a neighbourhood. Our experience is that despite a desire to be inclusive, the issue of interpretation is often fudged, particularly in small-scale evaluations. Even in larger studies there can be a gap between rhetoric and reality. Bhopal *et al.* (2004) reviewed UK studies on the prevalence of alcohol and tobacco in ethnic minority groups and examined whether they had met established guidelines for ensuring cross-cultural validity of questionnaires. Their analysis revealed that none of the surveys, including five national ones, had followed all of these guidelines.

Dilemma 2: Blending in

The second dilemma comes from an evaluation of a Health of Men project (White and Cash 2005) based on four case study sites: a barber's shop, a drop-in advice service, a youth centre and a council depot. The aim of the project was to improve access to health advice for men through provision of informal services. It was therefore essential that the evaluation, in seeking to examine the impact of the project on users, was carried out in a way that did not deter people from seeking advice in any way. An approach based on drop-in sessions and informal health advice meant that there was no register of service users which could have been used as a sample frame to select participants. There were additional issues around confidentiality and the need to prevent any embarrassment for men using the services. To overcome some of these issues, rather than relying on formal interviews or question-naires, the evaluators chose to use non-participant observation in the differ-ent settings to watch the interaction between the project workers and men. Short opportunistic interviews were planned but this turned out to more difficult than anticipated. In the youth centre, for example, the boys were boisterous and it was difficult to get them to concentrate. Some interviews were carried out in the council depot, but these were very limited because the men felt the need to get back to work. Despite the difficulties, the evaluation was successful at capturing the work of the Health of Men project through fieldnotes and records of informal conversations in the settings. A balance had to be struck between obtaining good data and not getting in the way of the work taking place. Failure to deal with this issue would have resulted in the evaluation posing an additional barrier to accessing health advice in those settings.

↻ Points for reflection

Does the notion of a balance between information needs and needs of partici-pants apply to any evaluation that you are familiar with?

Evaluation with hard-to-reach groups may mean that traditional research methods are neither practical nor appropriate. What other, less unobtrusive, methods can be used in such evaluations?

Dilemma 3: The outside perspective

The final example illustrates a common dilemma encountered when trying to capture the views of people outside a project or not in the know. The evaluation was investigating how a group of health trusts were involving local communities in planning and decision-making (South 2004). As part of the evaluation, key informants, such as lead managers, were sampled on the basis of personal involvement with the initiative. Naturally, these people were able to give in-depth responses about changes that had occurred. It was also important to obtain the views of people *not* engaged in that work to get a perspective on how the initiative related to mainstream activity. The dilemma was then whom to select, as it was important that respondents would feel comfortable talking about the topic but at the same time be able to give an 'outside' perspective. Quite often when individuals were approached, they found it difficult to understand why they were being asked for interview. In fact those interviews were vital to develop a holistic view of the initiative and confirm emerging findings.

This example shows the importance of involving people outside of a project as well as those in the know. The use of key informants is a common practice in evaluation, particularly where there are time or resource constraints. However, we need to recognize that such informants are often giving an internal perspective, which may paint a more positive picture than other stakeholders. The difficulty though for evaluators is being able to identify external voices and making sure their views are included. Stakeholders who are not directly involved in programme activity may feel that they have little to gain from taking part in an evaluation.

Points for reflection

How important is it to include the views of those not involved in an initiative? How easy is it?

How might you motivate them to participate?

The dilemmas described here illustrate just some of the many challenges facing evaluators in identifying and involving hard-to-reach groups. In the real world, such challenges are frequently met with limited resources which constrain responsiveness. Projects focused on specific communities of interest may be able to successfully engage participants in evaluation, but in more comprehensive programmes, decisions about who to involve and how to evaluate will be more problematic. In attempting to face up to some of the issues, evaluators may feel that they will be damned if they do and damned if they don't. Ultimately a balance needs to be struck which takes account of the aims and underpinning values of the initiative, the needs of different stakeholders, ethical concerns and methodological issues. The questions 'what is a good enough evaluation?', 'how can that be achieved?' and 'who will judge it?' need to be posed. There is a body of literature examining the conduct of research with vulnerable and marginalized groups, but the focus tends to be on academic studies. Overall there is a gap in the literature dealing with issues for evaluation and appraisal of practical, grounded strategies. In some fields this gap is closing as developments in policy and practice have stimulated discussion on valid approaches. For example, there is now a growing literature built on the experience of evaluation with children and young people (Swords 2002; Coad and Lewis 2004; Kirby 2004).

Strategies for evaluation with hard-to-reach groups

We now examine some of the strategies that can be adopted in evaluations with hard-to-reach groups. These should not, of course, be seen as technical fixes, rather as approaches that can be considered, depending on the context and purpose of the evaluation. Four key aspects are discussed:

- using participatory approaches;
- working with gatekeepers;
- sampling strategies;
- rethinking data collection.

The starting point, particularly where marginalized groups have been identified, should be good knowledge and understanding of the target population. Information about the profile and characteristics of a given community can be gathered from national statistics, local service data and from previous research or consultations (Gabbay and Gabby 1997). Local knowledge can also be gained through key informants such as local health professionals, community practitioners, community leaders and existing local groups. Such sources are particularly important in areas of high population mobility where official data rapidly becomes out of date. The different types of information can be then fed into evaluation planning and should inform selection of approaches and methods.

Using participatory approaches

In Chapter 5 we discussed the advantages and disadvantages of using participatory approaches for programme evaluation. Such approaches are particularly relevant for evaluation with vulnerable and hard-to-reach groups. Indeed, some would argue that participation in the research process is essential not simply for functional reasons but to redress inequalities and minimize the power imbalance between researchers and researched (Feuerstein 1986; De Koning and Martin 1996). Collaborating with community organizations allows evaluators to gain insider knowledge, to select appropriate designs and methods, and to identify practical access and sampling strategies. There are advantages in using researchers drawn from the same community, as cultural and language barriers to data collection and analysis can be minimized. Where there is hostility or fear of research, having peers involved in data collection helps reassure potential participants and may lead to greater willingness to disclose and discuss sensitive issues (Benoit et al. 2005). As indicated in Chapter 5, long-term investment in participation can build capacity in marginalized communities through developing the skills and experience of those involved. Box 7.1 provides an example of a successful collaborative project involving socially excluded youth as partners in designing and evaluating an intervention for reducing risk behaviours around HIV (Harper and Carver 1999). The authors conclude:

> Having true involvement from members of the target population can facilitate the conduct of such research with high-risk youth populations who are in desperate need of health education services but who are trad-

itionally suspicious of adults. These collaborative partnerships improve both the science and the service . . .

Using participatory approaches is certainly not without risk and should not be seen as a quick fix. Sullivan *et al.* (2001: 147) comment that: 'each project that fails to address community concerns further erodes the community's trust' – a point which all those involved in evaluation need to have constantly in mind.

Box 7.1 Involving street youth in evaluating an HIV prevention programme (Harper and Carver 1999)

The Youth Action Project was set up in a suburban area in California to investigate HIV risk behaviour in street youth and to evaluate prevention strategies. The project was run collaboratively between a university and a community-based organization, with young people actively involved from the beginning. High-risk street youth, such as teenagers who regularly truanted, were targeted. This was literally a hidden population as young people in the area were discouraged from loitering in public spaces. An initial survey of 677 young people was carried out to assess risk behaviours which informed the development of the programme. HIV prevention workshops for 277 young people were then evaluated using pre- and post-questionnaires administered over the course of a year. Young men and women from the target population were employed as youth outreach workers and received extensive training and support to undertake the evaluation. They were involved at all stages of the study, including:

- the study design and sampling
- development of relevant measures (which were translated into street language)
- recruitment of participants from sites where young people congregated
- data collection
- follow-up of participants
- designing youth-friendly educational materials.

The high level of involvement helped the project access this hard-to-reach group as youth outreach workers were able to overcome barriers and gain the trust of participants. This ultimately resulted in youth health needs being more visible and a credible prevention programme being supported and evaluated.

Working with gatekeepers

Much has been written about the role of gatekeepers in facilitating access to research populations. Gatekeepers can act as social and cultural guides and help with sampling and recruitment; this can be a valuable strategy for evaluations with hard-to-reach groups. Gatekeepers might include:

- community workers
- practitioners and managers from local services
- local teachers and school staff
- members of community and voluntary organizations
- faith and community leaders
- local politicians.

From the perspective of those being evaluated, gatekeepers can be a trusted and credible source of support, enabling individuals to take part in evaluation. Health projects working with disadvantaged groups frequently employ or work with people drawn from those communities. These individuals can be a valuable source of advice and act as gatekeepers. Indeed, in many cases, this will be the only way an evaluator will gain access to the target population. Where minority ethnic communities are involved, link workers can additionally provide language support (Gillam and Levenson 1999; Haour-Knipe *et al.* 1999).

Use of gatekeepers raises some specific issues for evaluation. A gatekeeper may feel a conflict of interest in enabling people to voice their views and at the same time trying to present the best possible perspective on a project, especially where evaluation is linked to continuation of funding. This may influence the selection of service users and the degree of access granted. Curtis *et al.* (2004) discuss some of the challenges of evaluating projects with hard-to-reach children and teenagers. One of the issues they raise is that project workers acting as gatekeepers may be keen to assist and encourage young people to take part but this can make fully informed consent difficult. Young people can find it harder to express dissenting views in those contexts, but at the same time they found that using staff members in focus groups provided essential support for young people when strong feelings arose or sensitive issues were discussed. We suspect that these are common issues; with hard-to-reach groups there is frequently a tension between project workers providing necessary support to allow people to take part in an evaluation and the possibility that participants will feel obliged to only report positive views. Another issue is that use of gatekeepers can widen participation in an evaluation but there needs to be recognition that representation from all sections of a community will not usually be achieved. Link workers may be the only practical solution to engage research participants, particularly where language barriers exist, but inevitably this limits access to those already in contact with services. Commissioning independent support, for example interpreters, as part of an evaluation is not always a viable option and may anyway fail to address barriers to participation. Overall, although use of gatekeepers is an effective strategy for evaluation with hard-to-reach groups, there are real challenges in trying to draw on the perspectives of those not using services or not in touch with key workers.

Sampling strategies

Sampling and recruiting individuals from hard-to-reach groups poses challenges, but adopting good sampling strategies can ensure that the evaluation includes views from all relevant groups. At the planning stage evaluators need to identify who they want to involve and what the issues are for sampling and recruitment. The utility of a sampling strategy will depend on its fit with the overall evaluation plan. For example, a sampling strategy for a project working directly with refugee families is likely to differ from that used for a service evaluation where the views of all local families, including refugees, are sought. Some of the issues for sampling hard-to-reach groups are as follows:

- the lack of a sample frame providing a list of potential participants – for example, homeless people are unlikely to be identified through official registers held by local services
- transient populations where sample frames are likely to be incomplete or out of date
- where there is insufficient information about the characteristics of individuals – for example, consider how an evaluation of a women's health initiative would draw up a sample to include lesbian women
- achieving representation when there are only small numbers of people
- groups where there is resistance to being identified, for legal reasons or because of stigma (Benoit *et al.* 2005).

Lee (1993), who has written extensively on research with vulnerable groups, suggests a number of sampling strategies for rare or 'deviant' populations (where people are outside the mainstream). Lee's seven methods are listed in Table 7.1 and we provide examples of how they might be applied in public health evaluation.

Evidently all the methods in Table 7.1 can be used for evaluation, but each one has its own limitations and can introduce considerable bias into a sample. Snowball sampling has gained a lot of credibility in public health research and can be particularly useful where mistrust towards statutory services has built up or where there are barriers to access. Lee (1993) points out that use of networks tends to give homogeneous samples, so there may still be people who are not included. McLean and Campbell (2003) discuss how wider social dynamics and the existence of networks influence recruitment from multi-ethnic communities. They recommend researchers use different sites and methods depending on the social context and also allow sufficient time. Lazenbatt *et al.* (2000: 86) point out that experimental designs preclude the use of community networks for recruitment, yet such networks are an essential part of a community-based practice. One further issue for evaluation is the potential for blurring between outreach activity and the process of sampling. Project workers or volunteers may have dual roles and the evaluation may result in an increased profile for a project in a given community (Haour-Knipe *et al.* 1999).

Table 7.1 Sampling methods for hard-to-reach groups

Sampling method	What it involves	Example
List sampling	Use of lists to identify individuals	Sampling Asian names from a general practitioner's register
Multi-purposing	Individuals are identified from the results of other surveys	A survey on local amenities giving a subsample of people with disabilities
Screening	The researcher casts a wide net and sifts through in order to pick up a few cases	Knocking on doors to identify older people at risk of social isolation
Snowball sampling	Use of networks where contacts identify other individuals known to them who in turn lead to more contacts	Asking sex workers to approach other women and men involved in similar work
Outcropping	Sampling through settings and groups where hard-to-reach populations meet	Using self-help organizations to sample carers
Advertising	Advertising for volunteers	Recruiting people from a Bangladeshi community through adverts on a community radio station
Servicing	Offering a service alongside the research	Working alongside an outreach project offering primary health care for the homeless

Source: Lee (1993).

Rethinking data collection

Given the limitations of commonly used methods, it is useful to think creatively and consider alternative methods of data collection. Common barriers to data collection include language, literacy and education barriers which make language-based methods problematic for some groups. Different cultural and social factors make some methods less acceptable or appealing, and this can affect engagement in the research process. Finally, there is the need to consider the potential for participants to feel threatened or disempowered by the process of data collection. Observational methods, both participant and non-participant observation, are very useful when working with marginalized groups where that type of power imbalance exists. The advantages are that observation can take place in natural settings, is usually less intrusive than questionnaires or interviews, and can be used where there are language barriers. Hurworth (2004) argues for the use of visual media, such as photography and videos, in programme evaluation. She suggests that such methods are useful in a number of contexts, including where:

- stakeholders are unable to participate in other forms of data collection – for example, evaluation with small children or with people with low literacy levels
- unobtrusive measures are required
- programme activity is itself highly visual, such as arts programmes
- the physical context or location is particularly important
- photography can be used by interactively in participatory evaluations.

There is growing interest in use of creative methods of evaluation, where data are collected, interpreted and the final product disseminated through an interactive process. This could be through visual arts, drama, music, or writing/narrative. Box 7.2 provides a wonderful example of where a creative evaluation was used successfully, enabling a group of women to record outcomes from their involvement in the project. Every picture tells a story and creative evaluations can potentially convey powerful messages about the effectiveness of a project; however, there are disadvantages in terms of ensuring rigour in analysis and how such evidence is viewed.

Box 7.2 Gardening for Health – a creative evaluation

Gardening for Health was an allotment project working with a group of non-English-speaking Bangladeshi women. The primary aims of the project were to address social isolation in this community and to help the women learn skills for growing fresh fruit and vegetables. The evaluation needed to capture the learning and other outcomes from the project, but a traditional approach with a written evaluation was deemed inappropriate. It was decided instead to use creative methods and base the evaluation on the production of a textile wall hanging. The women and project facilitators worked together using batik methods to produce panels illustrating what they had gained from the gardening project. The whole group then selected the final panels which one of the women made into a wall hanging. Up to 14 Bangladeshi women took part in the evaluation. Not only did the wall hanging provide a very tangible illustration of what had been gained from the project, but also the process of making and selecting the panels served as a tool for initiating conversations about what had been learnt, where things could be improved and ideas for future development. One of the advantages of the evaluation approach was that work on the wall hanging helped towards the aims of the project through building confidence and self-esteem. Following completion of the project, the wall hanging was successfully used for dissemination as a very visual way of celebrating what had been achieved. One facilitator also commented that the wall hanging was useful as a 'prop' to help the participants talk about what they had gained from the project.

There is evidently a need to look widely and if necessary move outside traditional evaluation paradigms, drawing on more creative and innovative methods as required. This is not to say that traditional approaches are never appropriate or that all research with hard-to-reach or vulnerable groups should be participatory and based on qualitative methods. Randomized controlled trials are possible with even the most vulnerable groups, but additional challenges may be present due to the reality of people's lives (Barlow *et al.* 2005). Evaluators using traditional approaches with hard-to-reach groups should bear in mind that the context and the needs of participants will have an impact on data collection and additional measures may need to be put in place to ensure inclusivity. Overall it is important to identify available options and to appraise their usefulness in the contexts of practice.

Measuring access and reach

Nutbeam (1998: 39) poses a key question for health promotion evaluation: did the programme reach the target population? He argues that it is necessary 'to determine the extent and level of exposure' to a programme in order to assess its effects. We have already touched on the importance of measuring reach. Effective programmes and projects will both use the right methods and reach the right people. Evaluation can highlight two common problems. The first is where programmes are working well but have limited coverage or lower levels of participation than anticipated. The second problem is where there is a mismatch between the actual and intended recipients. For example, a community project aimed at reducing social isolation may be well used and valued but may still fail to engage the most isolated individuals.

Two approaches can be used to assess reach. The more straightforward approach is to monitor referrals, contacts and uptake. Audit of monitoring data can then identify patterns of usage which can be compared to predictions based on target group characteristics. Monitoring and evaluating outreach services is more of a challenge because they are not static and it is more difficult to track individuals (Effective Interventions Unit 2002). An alternative approach to evaluating reach is to assess awareness of an initiative and reported use in the target population, for example, through a survey or community mapping. While this is a more resource-intensive approach, it may yield significant information on why people are not engaged.

Evaluation with hard-to-reach groups frequently involves grappling with the concept of access to health resources and services and how this can be measured. Access to health resources is evidently a central concern of both public health policy and practice, but there are debates on how access can be defined and measured and its relationship to concepts such as need, equity and coverage which are beyond the scope of this chapter (see Goddard and Smith 2001; Shengelia *et al.* 2005). For evaluation, the primary focus will not be on assessing health need but on finding out whether initiatives are meeting identified needs and how accessible they are. Gulliford *et al.* (2002) describe four dimensions for access to health care:

• service availability

- utilization of services and barriers to access
- relevance, effectiveness and access (if services are accessible then this will be reflected in health outcomes)
- equity of access.

We have identified how these might apply to evaluation of public health/ health promotion initiatives in Table 7.2. More often the approach to evaluating access is to look at utilization as a proxy indicator (Goddard and Smith 2001). In terms of practical strategies, projects can collect and analyse monitoring data on who uses services. If a project is accessible there should be some evidence that the profile of users reflects the diversity seen in the target population in terms of age, gender, ethnicity, area of residence and so on.

Table 7.2 Dimensions of access applied to evaluation of public health

Dimension of access	Application to public health	Example of indicators of access applied to a Walking for Health scheme
Service availability	Level of public health services/ activities provided	Numbers of local groups and frequency Walking groups held at a range of times and locations
Utilization of services and barriers to access	Utilization of public health programmes: • participation in health projects • participation in health-promoting activities • accessing health information or advice	Numbers of referrals Numbers attending walking scheme Register of participants reflects diversity in target communities in terms of age, ethnicity and gender Evidence that barriers to access have been addressed e.g. help with costs for public transport
Relevance, effectiveness and access	The extent to which public health programmes help people access health resources or enable people to have more control over their own health	Participants report the scheme has provided the right sort of support to enable them to increase their levels of physical activity
Equity of access	Public health programmes are responsive to different levels and types of health needs in individuals and communities	Evidence that the walking scheme has identified groups with specific needs in relation to physical activity and has adapted activities to ensure that they meet those needs Evidence that individuals from groups traditionally excluded from physical activity/leisure resources are able to take part in scheme

Monitoring utilization is not always straightforward. One of the early annual monitoring forms for Healthy Living Centres, for example, asked for data on numbers of users with disability and impairments including mental health problems or hidden conditions such as HIV/AIDS (where projects were targeting these groups). In treatment services this sort of information would be available but in community-based activities, such as drop-in groups, it presented a real challenge.

Monitoring data only gives a partial picture. There can be high levels of service utilization where there are limited choices in provision and it does not reveal the barriers to access that prevent people attending. Phillips *et al.* (1994: 161–3) suggest that accessibility should be evaluated across a number of aspects:

- access to goods and services, considering aspects such as distance, transport
- availability and approachability of service providers
- redress of grievances
- access to information
- access to decision-making processes.

The final case study illustrates a different and quite innovative approach to evaluating access across a number of criteria (Box 7.3). As we suggest in Chapter 8, what evaluators need to do is unpack what access might mean, which aspects they want to investigate, and identify some meaningful indicators.

Box 7.3 Undercover in Sheffield (Murray 2003)

The aim of this project was to get young people involved in evaluating sexual health clinics and outreach services using what was termed a 'mystery shopper' approach. The evaluation was based on the premise that young people's views and suggestions on services should be sought and should inform service development. Young people were recruited from schools, colleges and a youth project to take part in the evaluation. Eight women and two men aged 15–18 years undertook a training course to become 'undercover' evaluators. The mystery shopper approach involved the undercover evaluators making unannounced visits to services, presenting as a 'normal service user' and then assessing the service covertly. They recorded their observations and impressions against a number of criteria:

- accessing the service – both location and finding the service
- physical environment – the welcome given, atmosphere and whether the environment was youth-friendly
- confidentiality and the degree of privacy offered
- information – both the range and the methods of communication
- the reception area at clinics.

The evaluators were also asked to give their general impressions and to make suggestions for improvement. The visits were undertaken by different young people at different times to get a range of perspectives on each of the nine services assessed. Findings and recommendations were then summarized and the undercover evaluators were involved in feedback meetings with staff at each of the services.

Points for reflection

What were the advantages of recruiting a group of young people to evaluate these services?

What were the ethical implications for this evaluation?

Radical evaluation

Choices about evaluation are not made in a vacuum but within a broader political and moral framework and informed by the values of public health and health promotion. The wider theoretical debates on the nature of research and the exercise of power have relevance particularly where individuals or communities are disadvantaged (Holman 1987; Eakin et al. 1996; Truman et al. 2000). By failing to investigate the perspectives of marginalized groups, evaluations can perpetuate social exclusion. The voices of those most in need can be easily overlooked by default or even at times through discrimination. Paradoxically, even the ethical procedures put in place to protect disadvantaged groups can be so cumbersome that the outcome is increased barriers to participation. Additionally there is a tendency for research to focus on problems within communities rather than highlighting community strengths, thereby reinforcing negative stereotypes (Holman 1987; Eakin et al. 1996).

Critiques of power imbalances in traditional research have led to support for emancipatory and participatory approaches where research is linked to social action. Wallerstein points out, however, that intentions to use participatory approaches in evaluation do not always translate easily into practice and it is much harder to 'walk the talk' (1999: 40) than the literature often suggests. She argues that 'we have to be honest about our power-over bases in order to transform them to power-with the community' (1999: 49). An anti-exclusionary research framework would feature being explicit about the tensions that can arise (Truman et al. 2000). Smithies and Adams (1993) argue that evaluation should employ the principles of the new public health movement which would include consideration of equal opportunities policies in research methodologies. Most importantly, those engaged in evaluation with disadvantaged groups need some humility and sensitivity in their interaction with those who face oppression on a daily basis (Watson and Scraton 2001; Minkler 2004).

Evaluation, despite the challenges discussed so far, can be a powerful tool for change. Those involved in public health evaluation have responsibilities not only to funders and practitioners but also to the recipients of programmes and to the wider public. Evaluation that attempts to include the perspectives of the hard to reach can shed a light on inequities in provision. It provides evidence where initiatives effectively address health inequalities (Health Development Agency 2002). As all three case studies in this chapter show, it can facilitate people who are not often heard to voice their views be listened to. Witkin (2000: 211) argues that using a human rights approach means researchers 'help to articulate, illuminate and warrant' claims and 'provide a vehicle for their expression'. In these circumstances, evaluation can be radical in practice and be a mechanism for delivering genuine public accountability in public health programmes.

Summary

A variety of social, economic and cultural factors conspire to make some individuals and groups hard-to-reach. This has moral, ethical and methodological implications for the evaluation of universal health programmes and targeted initiatives working with specific groups. Throughout the chapter we have explored different strategies to involve hard-to-reach groups in evaluation. Some key themes are as follows:

- The social context and health needs of the target population should inform the selection of methods and sampling strategies.
- Participatory approaches working with community researchers can provide access to hard-to-reach populations.
- There needs to be more honesty and transparency in highlighting the difficulties and tensions in real-life evaluation situations.
- Programme reach and access to health resources are significant concepts and can be assessed from different perspectives.

8 | Measuring the fuzzy aspects

Overview

This chapter focuses on the challenge for evaluation in addressing some of the much used concepts within public health, which are open to different interpretations. It begins by considering these contested concepts and offers three different strategies for coping with them:

- identifying key constructs
- the use of frameworks and tools
- the use of narrative inquiry and story dialogue methods.

Contested concepts and evaluation

We have noted in earlier chapters that there are fundamentally important yet contested concepts within the field of public health, including the nature of health itself. There are also a number of terms, such as empowerment, community capacity, social capital and participation, which are interpreted differently by different groups and with varying degrees of precision. We collectively refer to these as 'fuzzy aspects', and they are characterized by:

- the absence of a universally agreed definition
- often being used loosely by practitioners to embrace different types of activity
- difficulty of measurement
- their central importance to public health
- the unclear distinction between their roles as instrumental or constitutive elements, that is, as means of achieving goals or as ends in themselves.

They present a particular challenge for evaluation. In this chapter we will consider possible approaches for dealing with these issues and propose alternative strategies. These include establishing conceptual clarity with regard to the focus of the evaluation and identifying key constructs as a basis for identifying indicators; using frameworks or tools to assist in measurement; and, drawing on an interpretivist perspective, using subjective interpretations. The strategies and approaches we refer to have been selected to provide insight into the process of disentangling complexity rather than as definitive solutions. We will draw on two principal themes to illustrate the approaches – empowerment and participation – but also make reference to related concepts such as social capital, community capacity and deprivation. Our commitment in writing this text was to avoid side-stepping the more challenging issues. These two themes both have the additional complication that, as well as being the focus of evaluation, they are also inextricably linked with the process of the evaluation itself. Evaluation can be participatory and/ or empowering, indeed, participatory and empowerment evaluation are both rapidly developing 'schools' of evaluation (see, for example, Fetterman and Wandersman 2005; Fetterman n.d.). However, for the purpose of this chapter, the focus on these issues is as the subject rather than the object of evaluation. We now turn to the first strategy.

Identifying key constructs

We noted in Chapter 3 that outcomes such as empowerment, participation and positive well-being offer particular challenges as regards measurement and yet they are of fundamental importance to public health and health promotion – as valued outcomes or the means of achieving them. Hubley (2002) comments that 'a disappointing feature of [his database on health promotion interventions in developing countries] has been the lack of published evaluations using either qualitative or quantitative research methodologies that demonstrate that empowerment has taken place'. He attributes this to 'the problematic and ill-defined nature of empowerment'.

Just as caricaturists attempt to capture their subject with a few deft strokes of the pen, evaluators need to be able to capture the essence of phenomena using a few well-chosen indicators. However, this should not be taken to belie the skill and familiarity with the concept required to make an appropriate selection. Furthermore, given the contested nature of these concepts, different evaluators may choose to give greater emphasis to some elements rather than others. The key issue is to make explicit the way the phenomenon of inquiry is conceptualized and what its basic constructs are held to be. In their review of methods for measuring deprivation, Carr-Hill and Chalmers-Dixon (2002) caution against the danger of the operational constructs of a phenomenon taking on the actual meaning of what they are held to represent – so-called reification. For example, the Jarman score, initially developed to identify the needs for primary care and as a basis for allocating additional payments to general practitioners, has, in the past, been widely adopted as a measure of area deprivation (Carstairs 1995). High Jarman UP8 scores became equated with deprivation even though they are not in themselves a comprehensive measure of deprivation. The more recent Index of Multiple Deprivation is broader and includes seven different domains, listed in Box 8.1. However, it should be borne in mind that, notwithstanding its more comprehensive remit, it remains an artificial construction of deprivation.

Box 8.1 English indices of deprivation, 2004

- Income deprivation
- Employment deprivation
- Health deprivation and disability
- Education, skills and training deprivation
- Barriers to housing and services
- Crime
- Living environment deprivation

Each domain contains a number of indicators. The criteria for inclusion of these indicators are that they should be 'domain specific' and appropriate for the purpose (as direct as possible measures of that form of deprivation); measuring major features of that deprivation (not conditions just experienced by a very small number of people or areas); up-to-date; capable of being updated on a regular basis; statistically robust; and available for the whole of England at a small area level in a consistent form. (Neighbourhood Renewal Unit 2004: 2)

Imposing some conceptual clarity on the 'fuzzy aspects' and breaking them down into key constructs makes measurement more feasible. For example, empowerment is frequently used in a rather general sense, but what exactly is being referred to – individual empowerment or community empowerment? How might they differ and what implications would this have for measurement? Furthermore, there is a distinction between the processes which lead to empowerment and empowerment itself. Reference to theory can help elucidate both the concept itself and its constructs.

Tones and Tilford (2001), for example, provide a useful analysis of self-empowerment in the context of health promotion. While a full discussion is not possible here, we will provide a simple overview to identify the implications for measurement. Self-empowerment is concerned with 'the genuine potential for making choices' (Tones and Green 2004: 35). At its core is the reciprocal relationship between individuals and their environment as shown in Figure 8.1.

The environment may facilitate or inhibit the capacity to make, express or achieve individual choice, and equally individuals may act to change their environment. The possession of appropriate health or life skills (such as communication, assertiveness and the ability to influence people and systems) will be necessary to achieve some control over environmental circumstances. While the environmental circumstances will ultimately determine the amount of control people actually have, **beliefs** about the control are a central feature of self-empowerment. These include perceived locus of control, which refers to an individual's general beliefs about whether consequences are the result of chance or fate (external locus) rather than the product of their own actions (internal locus). Self-efficacy beliefs are also

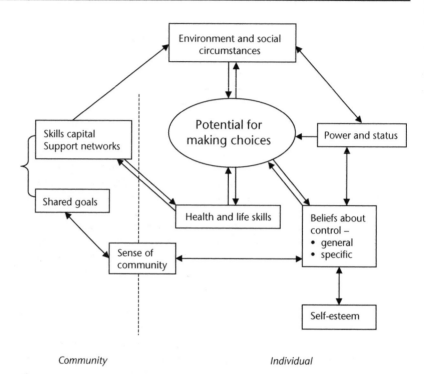

Figure 8.1 Empowerment

relevant. These are more specific and concern the belief that one is able to carry out specific actions. More general attributes such as self-esteem will contribute to beliefs about control and self-empowerment. Actual power and status will also have a direct bearing. It is worth noting the reciprocal relationship between many of the variables in Figure 8.1 – positive control together with requisite life skills will make it more likely that an individual will successfully take action, and the experience of so doing will further reinforce beliefs about control. Influences linked to the wider community, such as social support networks and sense of community, will also have some effect.

Having deconstructed empowerment, we can now apply it to developing indicators. Using the model as a reference point, each of the constructs of self-empowerment could be used to generate a series of relevant indicators. For example, a smoking cessation clinic based on empowerment principles might anticipate increasing self-efficacy beliefs in relation to stopping smoking, coping with any withdrawal symptoms, remaining smoke-free for a defined period, refusing the offer of a cigarette in a series of defined situations and so on. Similarly, the development of life skills might include assertiveness and stress management. Further examples for consideration are provided in Box 8.2.

Box 8.2 Unpacking the constructs of empowerment

The following initiatives could be based on empowerment principles:

- a school-based drop-in clinic for overweight young people
- a community initiative to lobby for the provision of a crossing patrol at a danger spot on a busy school route.

 Points for reflection

Suggest what self-efficacy beliefs and life skills might be expected to change as a result of these initiatives.

Alsop and Heinsohn (2005) provide a detailed account of how, working from a development perspective, they unpacked the concept of empowerment to produce a framework for measurement. Firstly, they offer a definition of empowerment as: 'enhancing an individual's or group's capacity to make choices and transform those choices into desired actions and outcomes' (Alsop and Heinsohn 2005: 5). They acknowledge that this includes both process and outcomes and proceed to then identify two main elements:

- personal agency, deriving from the ability to envisage options and make purposeful choices
- opportunity structure, the formal and informal contexts which make it more or less likely that choices will be put into action.

Following on from this, they identify indicators of agency, which are amenable to measurement. They refer to these collectively as asset endowments – psychological, informational, organizational, material, social, financial, or human. Table 8.1 gives proposed specific indicators for each. Similarly, opportunity structure is seen to derive from the existence and ways of working of both formal and informal institutions – including laws, regulatory frameworks and norms governing behaviour – and is similarly broken down into more detailed measures which can be adapted to suit different national, and indeed local, contexts. Although the various indicators offer different challenges for measurement and some will require mixed methods, breaking down the initially abstract concept into more concrete components opens up possibilities for the detailed specification of indicators and measurement.

However, the authors acknowledge that these are essentially antecedents of empowerment or 'intermediary indicators' (Alsop and Heinsohn 2005: 10) rather than empowerment itself. In addition to identifying the key contributing factors they also propose more direct measures:

- existence of choice
- use of choice
- achievement of choice

Table 8.1 Intermediate indicators of empowerment: agency

Asset base	Indicator
Psychological assets	Self-perceived exclusion from community activities
	Level of interaction/sociability with people from different social groups
	Capacity to envisage change, to aspire
Informational assets	Journey time to nearest working post office
	Journey time to nearest working telephone
	Frequency of radio listening
	Frequency of television watching
	Frequency of newspaper reading
	Passable road access to house (by periods of time)
	Perceived changes in access to information
	Completed education level
Organizational assets	Membership of organizations
	Effectiveness of group leadership
	Influence in selection of group leaders
	Level of diversity of group membership
Material assets	Land ownership
	Tool ownership
	Ownership of durable goods
	Type of housing
Financial assets	Employment history
	Level of indebtedness
	Sources of credit
	Household expenses
	Food expenditure
	Occupation
Human assets	Literacy levels
	Numeracy levels
	Health status

Source: Alsop and Heinsohn (2005: 63).

These levels of empowerment can exist at macro, intermediary, or local levels. For example, women in some countries may have considerable influence within families but little power at intermediary or macro levels. Furthermore, empowerment may be experienced differently within various domains. The authors identify three domains, each made up of subdomains as listed in Table 8.2. These are linked to the degree of empowerment at different levels by means of a framework. Agency and opportunity structure contribute to the experience of empowerment within each of the domains.

It will be evident that there are some similarities with Tones and Tilford's model, although Alsop and Heinsohn's emphasis is more towards external factors than the psychological constructs of empowerment. The key point is the necessity to be completely transparent about the way empowerment is conceptualized as a basis for evaluation and the development of a workable

Table 8.2 Levels of empowerment

		Degree of empowerment		
		Macro	Intermediary	Local
Domain	Subdomain			
State	Justice			
	Politics			
	Service delivery			
Market	Credit			
	Labor			
	Goods			
Society	Family			
	Community			

Source: adapted from Alsop and Heinsohn (2005).

model. An evaluation of the work of the Oxfam India Trust on women's empowerment (Oxfam 1999) focused on four key dimensions:

- capabilities – health and education enabling decision-making
- choices – opportunities available at various levels from family through to state
- assets – ownership and control of productive assets and property
- rights – the rights of women.

In all these examples the community has a mediating effect on individual agency. However, an empowered community is characterized by its capacity to take collective action – see Box 8.3.

Box 8.3 Definition of community empowerment

Community empowerment is 'a social action process in which individuals and groups act to gain mastery over their lives in the context of changing their social and political environment' (Wallerstein and Bernstein 1994: 142).

 Points for reflection

In what way/s does this differ from individual empowerment?

What implications does this have for measuring the process and outcomes of community empowerment?

Tones and Green (2004) identify the following key dimensions of an empowered community:

- a sense of community

- active commitment to achieving community goals
- high levels of social capital.

Each of these can be deconstructed to identify appropriate measures, but, by way of example, and given its current prominence, we will focus on social capital. Roberts and Roche (n.d.) encapsulate the problem of measuring social capital as

> measuring a phenomenon which is typified by abstract human relations such as trust, obligations and reciprocity in a way which, whilst remaining true to their complexities, reduces the level of abstraction in order to allow practical responses to be developed.

Their approach reflects that outlined above – identify key domains and produce indicators for each which can be 'captured' using either existing data sets or bespoke data-collection methods. The domains they identify are participation, altruism, trust and sociability. Clearly this approach could be adapted to suit the specific requirements of individual projects. However, it should be borne in mind that this fragmentation may fail to capture the essence of the whole.

There is inevitably some tension between developing specific local measures and using measures which are comparable across different areas. Harper and Kelly (2003) note the disparities in conceptualization and definitions of social capital and describe the approach taken by the Office for National Statistics Social Capital Project to achieve harmonization. The first stage was again to agree an operational definition, and after a detailed review the definition initially developed by OECD was adopted: 'networks together with shared norms, values and understandings that facilitate co-operation within or among groups' (Cote and Healy 2001: 41). Each element of the definition was then clarified. Following consideration of a number of different frameworks, the main dimensions for inclusion were identified (see Table 8.3) along with indicators and appropriate questions for use in surveys which are available on the National Statistics website, http://www.statistics.gov.uk/socialcapital/.

Point for reflection

Which of the indicators of social capital might be relevant to the evaluation of a local food co-operative?

The emphasis in this section has been on deconstructing concepts as a means of identifying relevant components, which can then be further operationalized into sets of indicators. Many frameworks derive from this type of theoretical analysis. We now turn our attention to the use of frameworks and tools.

Table 8.3 UK social capital measurement

Dimension	Examples of indicators
Social participation	Number of cultural, leisure, social groups belonged to and frequency and intensity of involvement Volunteering, frequency and intensity of involvement Religious activity
Civic participation	Perceptions of ability to influence events How well informed about local/national affairs Contact with public officials or political representatives Involvement with local action groups Propensity to vote
Social networks and social support	Frequency of seeing/speaking to relatives/friends/neighbours Extent of virtual networks and frequency of contact Number of close friends/relatives who live nearby Exchange of help Perceived control and satisfaction with life
Reciprocity and trust	Trust in other people who are like you Trust in other people who are not like you Confidence in institutions at different levels Doing favours and vice versa Perception of shared values
Views of the local area	Views on physical environment Facilities in the area Enjoyment of living in the area Fear of crime

Source: Harper and Kelly (2003: 7).

Using evaluation frameworks and tools

An alternative approach to measuring fuzzy aspects involves the use of evaluation frameworks and similar assessment tools. Like approaches based on unpacking key constructs, evaluation frameworks examine phenomena across a number of domains. The key difference is that instead of selecting from a menu of stand-alone indicators, frameworks provide integrated structures for evaluation and are usually accompanied by guidance on the processes of measurement. Their development can be seen to be a response to the need for practical 'off-the-shelf' resources to support robust evaluation in practice. Evaluation frameworks typically identify generic areas of measurement that can be adapted to local circumstances. We look now at the application of frameworks in evaluating participation and partnership working.

Participation is perhaps the ultimate fuzzy concept. Croft and Beresford

(1992: 20) point out that participation is 'one of those contentious words like "community" and "care" which can seem to mean everything and nothing'. Community participation is a central concept within public health, as both a valued goal and a mechanism for the achievement of other health-related goals. The plethora of terms in use (combinations of 'citizen', 'public', 'community', 'service user' and 'involvement', 'engagement', 'participation', 'partnership' are all used in current practice) in a sense reflects conceptual complexity and the diversity of practice. Any approach to the evaluation of participation requires clarity about goals, inputs and processes, in order to understand resulting outcomes. Barnes (1999) sets out six dimensions for analysis of participation:

- whose participation is being sought
- the type of knowledge to be accessed through participation
- the location within which participation is sought
- the objectives and purposes of participation
- the degree of power sharing
- the scope of participation and the level at which change is sought.

Understanding and defining what is being evaluated is a necessary first stage. This needs to be followed by questions relating to the quality and extent of participatory processes (how well are we doing?) and on outcomes (what has happened because of the participation?). Frameworks are useful here because they offer an integrative structure that can be applied at the different levels of a programme, from strategic planning through to single consultative activities, to produce answers to these questions.

Rifkin et al. (1988) developed one of the first frameworks for assessing participation in the context of Health for All and primary health care. Their work was based on an analysis of over one hundred case studies to identify factors influencing effective participation. The framework covers five areas: **needs assessment, leadership, organization, resource mobilization** and **management**. These are assessed on a continuum from narrow to wide participation and plotted on a spoke (visualization pentagram). The ranking scale was later simplified (Table 8.4) in an assessment of participation within a community-based accident prevention programme (Bjärås et al. 1991). Rifkin et al. (1988) suggest that the methodology allows differences to be assessed over time or between different stakeholders and facilitates learning in the programme.

The WHO Regional Office for Europe (1991) report on developing cross-national indicators for community involvement in health focused on public participation in health systems at local or district level. The final framework assesses participation using a series of questions grouped into four domains:

- effective communication and interaction between the community and the other parts of the health system
- representation of all sections of the community
- proper information as a basis for sound decision-making
- decision-making mechanisms which involve the community.

Table 8.4 Ranking scale for process indicators for community participation

Indicators	Narrow participation	Medium participation	Wide participation
Needs assessment	Professionals decide	Professionals and community define needs together	Community asks for programme
Leadership	Represents a small group of people	Combination of groups' interests	Represents many groups' interests
Organization	Rigid purpose, run by one or few organizations, run by professionals	In between	Flexibility in meeting goals; includes non-professionals
Resource mobilization	No contribution from beneficiaries	In between	Beneficiaries providing the major contribution
Management	External professionals make all decisions	Joint decisions by professionals and community	Community makes the decisions using professionals as resources

Source: Bjärås et al. (1991: 203).

In the UK a number of assessment tools for community statutory partnerships have been developed for use within different types of programmes (Markwell 2003). One that has been used extensively is a self-assessment tool for evaluating health alliances (Funnell et al. 1995). It contains sets of process and output indicators, and stakeholders are able to select appropriate indicators within generic categories, including community involvement. Like many similar evaluation frameworks, a set of questions, scoring mechanisms, exercises and guidance on how to complete an assessment are all provided. The focus of Funnell's tool is on the functioning of partnerships; however, it could be applied in a number of contexts where community involvement is sought. Hamer and Box (2000) describe how the tool was used successfully to evaluate involvement in a neighbourhood network. An alternative framework is *The Working Partnership*, a set of resources designed to assess partnerships and identify areas for improvement (Markwell et al. 2003). A series of questions are used to score different aspects on a scale of 0–5 for levels of action undertaken. Other relevant resources can be found from the field of regeneration. *Active Partners* (Yorkshire Forward 2000) is a framework based on ten benchmarks for participation, and *Auditing Public Participation* (Burns and Taylor 2000) is a practical evaluation resource with exercises and checklists to work through. To illustrate how frameworks and tools can be used to evaluate participation, we now describe some of the features of *Well Connected*, a self-assessment tool for community involvement.

Well Connected – an example of an assessment framework

Well Connected is a self-assessment tool for organizations on community involvement which emerged from work within Bradford Health Action Zone (Fairfax *et al.* 2002; South *et al.* 2005). The tool is designed to help organizations evaluate their progress against criteria in six key domains:

- *diversity* – whether community diversity is reflected in the organization and its processes
- *procedures* – whether organizational procedures facilitate participation
- *communication* – whether effective communication strategies are in place that allow flow of information between the organization and communities
- *staff support* – what the organization does to support and develop staff to engage with communities
- *opportunities* – whether communities are involved in the range of decision-making taking place in the organization
- *resources* – whether communities have access to and control of resources.

The tool uses a scoring system based on three elements: evidence of a strategic approach, good practice at different levels of the organization, and the range of opportunities and support available. An example of scoring for one of the criteria, in this case looking at how meetings and similar events are organized, is given in Table 8.5.

Table 8.5 Example of a ranking scale from *Well Connected*

	Score
The organisation has a strategic approach to organising meetings/events; processes are regularly reviewed and amended. Action is taken to minimise barriers to participation such as location, meeting style, procedures, timescales.	10
A range of styles/processes are used in meetings as appropriate. Some attention is given to barriers to participation but there is no strategic approach.	6–9
Some meetings/events are organised to facilitate participation – most are not; procedures and processes are not reviewed. Little attention is given to barriers to participation.	1–5
Meetings are barriers to participation, not thought about.	0

Source: Fairfax *et al.* (2002: 24).

The web, similar to other tools (Rifkin *et al.* 1988; Funnell *et al.* 1995), gives a visual representation of the assessment (see Figure 8.2). A fairly even shape in the outer areas of the web would indicate good community involvement. The initial assessment is then followed by a period where evidence is gathered from different sources. Examples of evidence include: policy documents, feedback from events involving communities, user surveys, community representation on committees, evidence of funding, and creation of specific posts working with communities. Gathering evidence allows organizations to validate the initial assessment and to see if there are any gaps between aspirations and the reality on the ground. The final stage involves revising scores, identifying areas for improvement and agreeing actions.

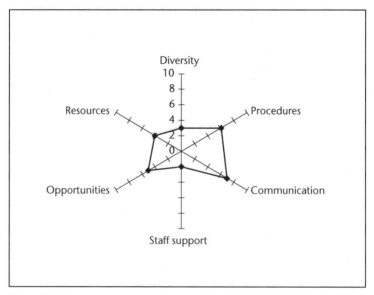

Figure 8.2 Example of a completed web

What can evaluation frameworks offer?

Evaluation frameworks have a number of strengths in relation to measuring fuzzy aspects such as participation. Firstly, they attempt to impose a structure and provide some clarity by identifying the core domains of measurement, thereby focusing data collection. In most cases these domains and the criteria for judgement have been derived either from empirical research or from extensive consultation with different stakeholders. For example, Funnell *et al.*'s (1995) tool was developed through extensive consultation and then piloted by practitioners working in health alliances. This bottom-up approach to identifying indicators and measurement domains gives the tools face validity and credibility in the field.

Secondly, evaluation frameworks can be used flexibly and applied to different settings and public health initiatives. In practice this allows evaluators to collect the most relevant evidence, depending on the context. What is perhaps more significant for fuzzy aspects is that frameworks, through using generic domains in a flexible way, are able to cope with the diversity of activities and actors. For example, Rifkin *et al.*'s (1988) indicator on leadership could be applied to a small community project as well as to a large community-wide programme with multiple levels of involvement.

Thirdly, many frameworks provide practitioners with a unified package of evaluation resources. Assessment processes are often based on reflection, discussion and learning in order to tease out qualitative aspects of participation and what it means to stakeholders. Quantitative measures or simplistic recording of activities tend not to be used. Concerns about 'tokenism' in participation mean that there should be an in-depth analysis of what is occurring, not just reliance on tick-boxes. There is an emphasis in many frameworks on the evaluation process, so it is not a static 'once and for all' assessment but rather a way to facilitate shared understandings and learning. This is another strength if programmes want to use evaluation tools to improve practice. For example, *The Working Partnership* (Markwell *et al.* 2003) helps organizations to identify future actions.

Evaluation frameworks may appear a good solution to measuring fuzzy aspects, somewhere between a theoretically driven approach and an interpretivist one. However, there remain measurement issues, including the question of objectivity. All of the tools reviewed above seek to draw on different sources of evidence and involve different stakeholders. Multiple perspectives on participation may not lead to a consensus – for example, there may be differences in ranking. The question of who is invited to participate in the assessment of criteria would need to be made explicit in reporting results.

The inherent flexibility of frameworks means that assessment results have limited comparability across programmes, whereas some of the standardized indicators do allow for comparison. There seems to be a tension between setting out clear indicators that get behind the fog of rhetoric and defining some of the fuzzy aspects too narrowly. This was certainly a tension in the development of *Well Connected*. Many of those consulted during the development phase welcomed more detail about what was being measured, but there was a risk that the tool would end up being too prescriptive and narrow in focus (South *et al.* 2005). To give an example, a narrowly focused indicator might be whether there were community representatives on a project board. In contrast, a more flexible approach would examine how well structures in a health project enabled community views to be heard.

Finally, in many of the frameworks for partnership working and participation there is an emphasis on investigating processes rather than outcomes. The evidence base on impact of community participation is weak precisely because it is difficult to attribute outcomes to what is a complex social process. A systematic review on community involvement in area-based initiatives noted that few studies used quantitative measures or examined the costs and benefits of involvement (Burton *et al.* 2004). El Ansari *et al.* (2001) discuss the nature of evidence in partnerships and acknowledge the difficulties of measurement and the multiple perspectives involved. They recommend more precision in relation to evaluation choices, such as whether short- or long-term effects are measured. While some might argue that an interpretive approach is more successful at drawing out outcomes for individuals, there is still a search for the holy grail of valid outcome measures for community participation.

The use of narrative inquiry and story dialogue methods

The assumption underpinning the foregoing has been that it is both possible and desirable to objectively measure these elusive concepts. While not wishing to re-engage in the epistemological debates referred to in Chapter 2, it is worth making a few points. The ability to 'measure' these complex concepts will allow evaluations to address them meaningfully and the evidence base to be built on how best to achieve these fundamental and valued goals. The question remains, however, whether it is feasible to accurately represent phenomena. The answer will be influenced by the rigour and transparency of the approach used, and we have provided some examples of how this might be achieved. Nonetheless, from an interpretivist position the quest is rather like chasing rainbows. The use of qualitative methods such as key stakeholder interviews, either alone or in conjunction with quantitative approaches, is held to provide 'illuminative insight' into processes and, indeed, the achievement of outcomes. Whatever evaluation strategy is adopted, it acts rather like a lens throwing some aspects of a programme into sharp relief while leaving others out of focus – and truly 'fuzzy'. Judgements about what to focus on will inevitably be shaped to an extent by the preconceptions and interests of those involved in designing the evaluation. The tendency for evaluations to focus on outcomes rather than process and context is well recognized. The complex causal web linking inputs and outcomes also receives little attention. Furthermore, Riley and Hawe (2005: 226) note that we hear little about the 'private contexts of practice' and, we might add, the private accounts of how interventions are received and affect target groups and populations. The challenge is how to capture these facets and the often unanticipated aspects of process and outcomes. We will conclude this chapter by considering the use of stories and narrative inquiry as one alternative strategy, which can provide access to these private accounts and subjective interpretations.

'Stories provide a forum for a process of describing, explaining and reflecting on how change has occurred' (Ontario Clearing House n.d.). The analysis of stories avoids fragmenting and decontextualizing the experiences of both providers and recipients of programmes. As Ashdown (n.d.: 5) notes: 'By listening to people together telling their story, the heart and soul of the project is revealed'. He notes the particular applicability to grassroots projects which often focus on producing results by 'get[ting] on with doing what they are doing rather than rigorous monitoring and assessment of outcomes' (Ashdown n.d.: 6). However, stories are equally applicable to large-scale projects and can complement qualitative and quantitative data – see, for example, the work in Australia of the Narrative Evaluation Action Research project:

Narrative can be an effective method of 're-chunking' rich, complex life back into a manageable way of understanding the bigger picture of more complex realities. The meanings of more abstracted quantitative and qualitative datasets can then also be more effectively understood. (Wadsworth *et al.* 2004: 6)

A selection of real 'stories' of people who have benefited from local community health centres in Toronto is provided at http://testweb.opc.on.ca/realstories/etext/sto.html – see Box 8.4 for brief extracts from two of these stories.

Box 8.4 Stories

Power

'In this community, most of the residents aren't politically active. They don't understand the system, they don't believe in the system and they don't think their vote counts. . . . We want to make sure that we get someone in there who is accountable to us,' says Dineen. 'Currently, because of the lack of vote at Regent Park, we don't have a lot of political power.'. . .

Walsh, Mintz and Dineen all say that the work is exhausting: fighting bureaucrats can be a daunting experience, particularly when the results seem to come slowly. But Regent Park residents have built themselves a strong community and they aren't about to roll over. 'We've all had traumatic things happen in our lives,' says Walsh. 'It's been tough for a lot of people in this community. The constant grind can grind you down. As far as fighting for our rights goes, well, our energy right now is low but we still don't give up.'

She says the voter education drive is just one small step in getting people to feel like they have enough power to change things around them. 'Some people say you can't do this but I know we can.' (http://testweb.opc.on.ca/realstories/findingpower.html)

Margo's story – Margo has MS

Most of us learn to take for granted the frustrations of dealing with the regular health care system . . . the long waits, the rushed visits, the constant shuffling among specialists who only know or care to know one small part of you, the feeling that you are little more than a collection of symptoms in need of medicinal solutions. From my very first contact with the Barrier Free Health Zone at The Station, a community health center in North Toronto, I realized that things *can* be different.

As I passed through the doors, the first feeling that struck me was ease. I breathed easily and felt so much more relaxed as I didn't have to maneuver around obstacles, cope with uneven floor spaces or deal with elevators and washrooms in which my scooter would not fit. Instantly, I felt as if this was a place outside of my constant efforts at having to adapt. Here was a place designed and adapted for *me*. (http://testweb.opc.on.ca/realstories/special.html)

↻ Point for reflection

What issues emerge from these stories that might have been overlooked using other strategies for data collection?

Stories can take many forms, both written and oral, and should include consideration of failures as well as successes. The characteristics of a 'good' story are summarized in Box 8.5.

Box 8.5 A good story

In the context of evaluation a good story is one which:

- demonstrates success or failure
- was particularly stimulating or perplexing for others
- offers some useful lessons or insights
- provides descriptive detail – who was involved, what actions took place, when and where, what went smoothly and what was problematic?
- gives reasons for actions – what issue was being addressed and why was it selected, how did actions produce change and how did organizational (or other) structures and relationships influence which actions were selected?
- leads to reflection – was there consensus or disagreement about action, with the benefit of experience what would you do differently and why?

Source: adapted from Ontario Clearing House (n.d.).

Punch (2005: 218) describes narratives as 'social constructions located within power structures and social milieux'. Although the terms 'story' and 'narrative' are often used interchangeably, Riley and Hawe (2005) make the distinction that people tell stories, but the narrative emerges from the analysis of these stories. While they acknowledge different approaches to narrative analysis, they identify two key features which distinguish it from other forms of qualitative analysis. Firstly, time and context influence the construction of meaning, and the past and future may co-exist with the present in the mind of the narrator. Secondly, the position of the narrator is central and other individuals – the supporting cast – are seen in relation to them. Riley and Hawe provide a detailed account of how they analysed the diaries kept for two years by community development officers working on a community development initiative with recent mothers. This involved the following steps:

- Examination of narrative segments – and assessment of whether they are descriptive, consequential (identifying cause–consequence links), evaluative (revealing attitudes) or transformative (involving a change in how the narrator sees things)
- Understanding why the story is being told in the way it is
- Examination of the storytelling occasion and the construction of the story in relation to the narrator, the listener/s and the context in which the story is told
- Exploration of how the process of meaning interacts with other norms or events
- Identifying the point of the story.

In response to frustrations that research and evaluation did not equate with the ' "reality" of practice', Labonte *et al.* (1999) worked in partnership with practitioners to develop a story/dialogue method suitable for a range of different purposes, including evaluation. The authors use their structured storytelling approach in a group context and contend that 'as stories are shared between people, they become "generative themes" for group reflection, analysis and action planning' (p. 40). The stories engage people in dialogue and provide the basis for further probing and analysis. Personal authority gives way to shared understanding within the group. The method involves developing and sharing case stories on chosen themes. There are two or three rounds of storytelling, each followed by reflection and structured dialogue using questions such as:

- What do you see happening here?
- Why do you think it happens?
- So what have we learned from our own experiences?
- Now what can we do about it?

The analysis is therefore interwoven with the rounds of storytelling and is based on the developing insights of those involved rather than an external agent. Each round of storytelling concludes with the production of 'in-sight cards' that contain the key points for action which have emerged. The method initially focuses on specific individual stories, but progressively 'metamorphoses' into lessons applicable to all practitioners and more abstract generalizations. It is able to cope with the complexity of change and the effect of contextual factors. Furthermore, it allows outcomes and processes which are of value to participants to emerge prominently.

Summary

We have presented two diametrically different approaches to coping with the 'fuzzy aspects' of evaluation: the use of theory to deconstruct key concepts, and the use of story and narrative to build up holistic interpretations.

Frameworks occupy some intermediary position. The choice will be up to practitioners, bearing in mind the respective advantages and disadvantages of each approach. However, common features of all three strategies are as follows:

- They acknowledge the complexity of practice and the contestability of major concepts in public health and health promotion.
- They seek to provide clarity for complex phenomena.
- They draw on multiple perspectives and different sources of evidence.

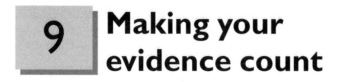

9 Making your evidence count

Overview

This chapter deals with an essential component of the evidence-based practice cycle – reporting and disseminating evaluation findings. It includes:

- the importance of dissemination
- reporting findings in ways which are relevant and convincing
- dissemination strategy
- the wider picture.

The importance of dissemination

The primary purpose of conducting evaluations is to inform decisions relating to either to the future direction of the project itself or the wider development of policy and practice. Furthermore, the move towards evidence-based practice is based on having access to evaluation evidence. It is essential, therefore, that evaluation findings are properly disseminated. A useful starting point is to consider your own use of evaluation findings.

 Points for reflection

Consider evaluation reports or journal articles that you are aware of.

How did you get to know about them?

How clearly were the findings communicated?

How relevant were they to you?

How convinced were you by the findings?

How useful were the findings in influencing practice or policy?

Dissemination has been defined as 'the active, purposeful process of knowledge transfer. Like evaluation processes, dissemination requires resources, infrastructure and planning and is essential in the feedback link to informing future planning' (Department of Human Services 2005). However, it is well recognized that little attention has been paid to the issue of dissemination of evaluation findings and the diffusion and maintenance of successful interventions. The evaluation task is often seen as complete with the publication of the final report. Time and budgetary constraints all too often get in the way of serious attempts to disseminate findings further and stem from lack of attention to this important aspect in the planning and commissioning of evaluations. As Johnson *et al.* (1996) note, 'The gap between knowledge generation and knowledge use or application remains problematic' (cited by Oldenburg *et al.* 1999: 121).

The focus of much evaluation is on what does or does not work rather than the factors that contributed to success, how these can be replicated and sustained and the diffusion and take-up of new ideas and ways of working. Oldenburg *et al.* (1999) audited articles appearing in 12 health promotion and public health journals during one calendar year. Of the 1210 articles identified, 39.5 per cent were concerned with health promotion research, and the focus of these was research and development 86% (of which 16% were interventions-based), innovation and development 5%, diffusion research 1.3%, and institutionalization research 6.3%.

A review of strategies for transferring knowledge into practice (NHS Centre for Reviews and Dissemination 1999) concluded that knowledge alone is unlikely to bring about change in professional practice or policy. In the same way that knowledge does not bring about change in health behaviour, simply making information available to practitioners does not mean that it will necessarily be acted on. Such change requires analysis of the various facilitating factors and barriers at individual, organizational and policy level. Change processes can usefully draw on relevant theory – learning theory, social cognition theory, diffusion and organizational change theory. Diffusion of innovations theory (Rogers and Shoemaker 1971; Rogers 1995), for example, indicates that the take-up of new ideas and practices is usually slow in the first instance, involving so-called innovators and early adopters. It then gathers pace as the early and late majority come on board, before finally slowing down when only those most resistant to change – the laggards – remain (see Figure 3.1). According to Tones and Green (2004), over and above the characteristics of the adopters themselves, a number of other factors influence the overall rate of change:

- the nature of the social system
- the channel for communication
- the perceived characteristics of the innovation – including relative advantage and compatibility with existing practice
- leadership and the role of change agents
- participation.

A discussion of the multiplicity of factors involved in achieving change in policy or practice is beyond the remit of this text. However, the dissemination of research and evaluation evidence through appropriate channels to reach key decision-makers and opinion leaders is a crucial first stage in raising awareness of important findings. If evaluation research is to provide a secure basis for decision-making at micro or macro level, then attention will need to be given to the quality of evaluation reports and the strategy used for communicating findings to different stakeholder groups. This chapter will address the challenges associated with publication and dissemination of findings. It will begin by considering ways of reporting evaluation findings and identify what should be included in evaluation reports to maximize their utility. It will then look at the dissemination strategy and the more general relevance of individual evaluations to evidence-based practice.

Reporting findings

While, conventionally, evaluation findings are presented in full in a written report, alternative formats are possible and, indeed, in many instances desirable (see Box 9.1). In addition to traditional print media we are witnessing an increase in the use of electronic media and dissemination via websites. McNeish and Downie (n.d.) emphasize the importance of considering translation into minority languages and the use of large-print and Braille versions.

Box 9.1 Types of evaluation report

Full written report
Summaries for different stakeholder groups
Electronic web-based reports
Verbal presentations
Workshops/presentations for practitioners
Seminars
Conference presentations
Journal articles: professional journals; academic peer-reviewed journals
Newsletters
Media – newspapers, radio, television
Posters
Visual displays
Video

Points for reflection

What would be the advantages and disadvantages of these various formats for different groups?

Which would be most appropriate for communicating findings to marginalized groups?

A formal written report is usually required by project funders or managers and commissioners of evaluation and will provide a complete and permanent record of the evaluation process and findings. However, many users of evaluation will have neither the time nor the inclination to read lengthy reports. Providing executive summaries and other brief targeted summaries for key stakeholder groups will assist in communicating findings to a wider audience. The acronym KISS is often used to encapsulate how best to communicate information to politicians – Keep It Short and Simple – but is equally applicable to other groups. Having a clear view of the purpose of reporting will help in identifying the most appropriate medium, style and content. For example, is it to inform practice within the project or organization or contribute to the wider evidence base? Is it intended to persuade funders or to influence micro- or macro-level policy? Is it to gain maximum publicity for any achievements? Evaluators frequently publish findings in academic journals, yet many practitioners find the terminology and/or the style of these inaccessible (Barnardo's Research and Development Team 2000). Alternative media, including direct mailing or invited seminars, may be more effective ways of reaching them.

The *Framework for Program Evaluation in Public Health* of the Centres for Disease Control and Prevention (Milstein and Wetterhall 1999) notes that 'Regardless of how communications are constructed, the goal for dissemination is to achieve full disclosure and impartial reporting'. The Framework provides a checklist of items adapted from Worthen *et al.* (1996) to make evaluation reporting more effective.

- Provide interim and final reports to intended users in time for use.
- Tailor the report content, format, and style for the audience(s) by involving audience members.
- Include a summary.
- Summarize the description of the stakeholders and how they were engaged.
- Describe essential features of the program (e.g. including logic models).
- Explain the focus of the evaluation and its limitations.
- Include an adequate summary of the evaluation plan and procedures.
- Provide all necessary technical information (e.g. in appendices).
- Specify the standards and criteria for evaluative judgments.
- Explain the evaluative judgments and how they are supported by the evidence.
- List both strengths and weaknesses of the evaluation.
- Discuss recommendations for action with their advantages, disadvantages, and resource implications.
- Ensure protections for program clients and other stakeholders.
- Anticipate how people or organizations might be affected by the findings.
- Present minority opinions or rejoinders where necessary.
- Verify that the report is accurate and unbiased.
- Organize the report logically and include appropriate details.
- Remove technical jargon.
- Use examples, illustrations, graphics, and stories. (Milstein and Wetterhall 1999: Box 11)

Being relevant and convincing

We have considered at some length in earlier chapters various approaches to gathering evaluation evidence. Reporting findings requires both analysis and interpretation of the data collected and the development of conclusions and recommendations. The critical appraisal tool developed by the Health Development Agency (Swann *et al.* 2005) for assessing the quality of review papers for inclusion within its evidence base also provides useful pointers for those writing evaluation reports. Key considerations include:

- systematicity
- transparency
- quality
- relevance.

Quality and systematicity apply to the evaluation process itself as well as the way that it is reported. Evaluation reports should also be transparent about the methods used and the rationale for using them, any values implicit in the evaluation and the basis for reaching conclusions about what has or has not been achieved. Ultimately, the utility of the findings will depend on their relevance to key stakeholder groups. A theme running through this text has been the importance of involving key stakeholders throughout the evaluation process in order to understand their needs and ensure that they are addressed by the evaluation. The *Framework for Program Evaluation in Public Health* notes that:

> When stakeholders are not engaged, an evaluation might not address important elements of a program's objectives, operations and outcomes. Therefore, evaluation findings might be ignored, criticized, or resisted because the evaluation did not address the stakeholders' concerns or values. (Milstein and Wetterhall 1999)

It identifies the following categories of key stakeholders:

- those involved in program operations (e.g., sponsors, collaborators, coalition partners, funding officials, administrators, managers, and staff)
- those served or affected by the program (e.g., clients, family members, neighborhood organizations, academic institutions, elected officials, advocacy groups, professional associations, skeptics, opponents, and staff of related or competing organizations)
- primary users of the evaluation.

Relevance can also be linked to timing. Interest is always greatest when findings are applicable to current priorities or needs. However, the time schedule for reporting evaluation findings may be dictated by external agendas and political factors rather than the natural cycle of research and development. Pawson (2002: 340) notes that the 'policy cycle revolves more quickly than the research cycle'. It is not unusual for programmes to be required to report evaluation findings at too early a stage in their development, and well before some of the anticipated effects can be expected to emerge – see the case study in Box 9.2.

Box 9.2 Dissemination case study

In September 2005, newspaper headlines carried the message that Sure Start, the government programme for families of children under 4, was failing. A leaked report showed that there was little difference for children in Sure Start Local Programme areas compared with non-Sure Start areas. At the time of the leak, it was suggested that there was considerable political pressure to report the early results due to a change in government policy. When the actual research report was published some two months later, it presented a more complex picture of both negative and positive change across a number of aspects of parenting and child development, although in all cases the size of the effect was small (NESS Team 2005). The report pointed out that these results could only give an early indication of impact as research had shown that local programmes usually took three years before they were delivering the full range of services. One editorial put the disappointing results in perspective: 'The research findings should not come as a surprise. It was the equivalent of the under-fives pulling up recently sown radishes to see if their vegetables were growing' (*Guardian* 2005).

Although a national study, it is worth considering the issues for dissemination in this example. It is not unusual for evaluations to have to feed results into decision-making processes before projects have had time to become fully established. More often this is not because of a perverse desire to see projects fail but because the political will to address health problems drives both the need for information and speed in wider implementation. The National Sure Start Evaluation will continue to follow children up over time, but it is common that small-scale evaluations are not funded to measure outcomes over a sufficient period of time to see changes in health behaviour or health status. This raises questions about how results are reported and disseminated. It is important to strike a balance between identifying firm evidence relating to outcomes and not setting up projects to fail. There are additional issues, as in the case study, of how key messages can be reported on without losing the complexity of the findings. In the worse cases those involved in the evaluation may lose control of results and find new meanings assigned to their data.

Points for reflection

Thinking about the analogy of children's impatience at waiting for seeds to grow, identify any examples where evaluation was conducted too soon to adequately capture the outcomes or where there was insufficient time for learning to be fed back.

What can be done to address these issues?

What reporting strategies can be used to prevent misinterpretation and promote good understanding of the findings?

Most published research, as we noted earlier, tends to be more concerned with outcomes than with the process of programme delivery and the identification of those factors which are critical to success. Yet for practitioners seeking to replicate achievements or for those concerned with policy development, this is of primary interest – a point we will return to later. 'Unfortunately, however, the critical information required for judging both the quality of a public health intervention and whether or not an intervention is worthwhile or replicable is missing for most public health intervention studies' (Jackson and Waters 2005: 367). It is essential, therefore, that evaluators report this information. Barry *et al.* (2005: 31) propose that the following aspects should be included:

- programme adherence or fidelity
- exposure
- quality of programme delivery
- participant responsiveness
- programme differentiation.

A major challenge when reporting findings is how to capture significant and at times life-changing outcomes, or alternatively moments of breakthrough in getting programmes up and running. The media and politicians have long recognized the power of the human story, yet evaluators, in pursuit of objectivity, have tended to ignore it and direct their attention more to community or population change. By doing so, what might amount to substantial change among a few individuals can easily become averaged out among the target population as a whole. Case studies can be used to redress this problem and add illuminative insight to evaluation reports about both the real experiences of practitioners and recipients of the programme. One innovative approach to conveying the way in which a programme works, how it has been successful and how others might replicate it, has been through the use of 'success stories' based on the North Carolina *Community Change Chronicles*. The WISEWOMAN project (Lewis *et al.* 2004), administered by the CDC, involves 14 demonstration projects which aim to reduce heart disease, stroke and other chronic disease in uninsured women in the USA. While longer-term goals are concerned with disease reduction, the project has used stories as a means of identifying more immediate outcomes and communicating findings to policy-makers and public health professionals. The stories are written to a common format that includes:

- Title – which conveys the purpose of the intervention
- Statement of need – identifying the particular public health problem addressed
- Project details – which include process information
- Main results – which summarizes anticipated and unanticipated successes among the women who participated and community partners as well as on the part of project staff
- Lessons learned – which identifies key elements that led to success and also what did not work.

Two volumes of compilations of these stories have been published (Centers for Disease Control and Prevention 2003, 2005). The stories have been used extensively in dissemination – for example, to educate staff, share lessons learned, raise awareness of opportunities and how to realize them, inform politicians and other decision-makers, as well as to publicize success and acknowledge the contributions of partners. This approach is held to be particularly effective because it puts 'a human face on a project's challenges and achievements' (Lewis *et al.* 2004: 617). It also describes achievements and processes not readily captured by more conventional methods which rely on aggregation of findings.

Dissemination strategy

A fundamental question for evaluators is where their responsibility for dissemination ends. Rather than being an end in itself, the production of the evaluation report, in whatever form, should be the first stage in informing future decision-making. The dissemination strategy needs to go beyond mere consideration of how many copies of reports need to be produced, in what format and for which groups, to address how the findings can be put to best use. Clearly, if dissemination is to be taken seriously, then it needs to be properly planned and resourced, formally included in the evaluation design and, indeed, specified in the commissioning process for external evaluations.

In the first instance, the practical implications for the project itself and the immediate stakeholders need to be specified and fed back in the most appropriate way. However, the findings may also be relevant to the wider community of public health practitioners, policy-makers and academics. This wider dissemination may be seen as an obligation for major demonstration projects and publicly funded evaluations. However, small-scale projects often do not recognize the relevance of their work to others. As a result, many potentially useful evaluation reports of interventions carried out under everyday circumstances and in the real world remain lost in the so-called 'grey literature'. If they are to be brought to the attention of this wider community then the dissemination strategy will need to consider publication in some form within the public domain. Those involved in small-scale evaluations can feel deterred from seeking wider dissemination for two main reasons, over and above any lack of experience in publication and resources to allocate to the task. Firstly, small-scale evaluations have limited external validity. Secondly, it is often difficult to demonstrate significant change at the small-group level. However, the process of programme implementation and the causal pathways of change can often be unpicked more easily at the smaller scale, drawing on some of the methodological approaches we described earlier. The orientation of small-scale evaluation reports could therefore be towards this aspect rather than whether an intervention works or not. An overview of what to include in evaluation reports of small projects is provided in Box 9.3.

Box 9.3 A template for reporting small projects

Introduction

Background to the project and the problem/issue it aims to address; aims and objectives and theory of change; summary of the main activities and resources; details about the target population; information about the context.

Evaluation methods

Description of the evaluation approach, data-collection methods and sampling (applied to both process and outcomes); any limitations of the evaluation; any problems with data collection.

Findings

The main findings about the delivery of the project, including barriers, facilitating factors and context, and any evidence about success. If there are a number of different components to the project, it may be necessary to present the findings for each separately.

Discussion

(i) *Lessons learned:* what has been learned about good practice which could be transferred to other projects or situations; with the benefit of hindsight, what would be done the same and what would be done differently.

(ii) *Key issues to emerge:* what do the findings reveal about achievements or lack thereof; what particular aspects of the way the project was delivered or the context contributed to this; whether any groups benefit to a greater extent than others and why; what are the strengths and weaknesses of the project; what are the major challenges in rolling this project out further that may be of relevance to managers and commissioners.

Conclusions and recommendations

Summary of the key point to emerge; concise recommendations which have emerged from the findings.

Rychetnik and Wise (2004: 252) found that

> an important message from both the literature and our own discussions
> with policy makers is that research findings will rarely speak for them-
> selves. Health promotion advocates who are experienced lobbyists, regular
> policy advisors or policy makers themselves all live and breathe by this
> principle.

They also note the reluctance to communicate the practical implications of
research, let alone becoming actively involved in advocacy and lobbying.
This they attribute to

- scientific conservatism and unwillingness to go beyond the 'demonstrated facts';
- maintaining credibility as an objective, independent researcher;
- lack of experience and training in how to influence public health policy
  and practice.

Further, even when researchers do make recommendations about policy or
practice, they are frequently not grounded in practical and political realities.

Research by Barnardo's Research and Development Team (2000) for the
Joseph Rowntree Foundation looked at the views of key stakeholders in
research – commissioners, researchers, disseminators and users – about how
research findings in the social welfare field could best be integrated into
practice. The key factor to emerge was allocating dedicated resources to
dissemination. Their suggestions for issues that should be considered for
improving dissemination are listed below. In particular, the list emphasizes
those areas that researchers/academics should be aware of to ensure that their
findings are published and used. For commissioners they suggest:

- Timing
- Relevance to the current policy agenda
- Allocating dedicated development resources within research funding
- Including a clear dissemination strategy at the outset
- Involving professional research users in the commissioning process
- Involving service users in the research
- Commissioning research reviews to synthesize and evaluate research.

For researchers the list of suggestions is as follows:

- Provide accessible summaries of research.
- Keep the research report brief and concise.
- Publish in journals or publications which are user-friendly.
- Use language and styles of presentation which engage interest.
- Target the material to the needs of the audience – policy-makers and
  managers preferred bullet-point summaries, whereas practitioners and
  service users valued verbal feedback.
- Extract the policy and practice implications of research – ideally in part-
  nership with practitioners and policy-makers.
- Tailor dissemination events to the target audience and evaluate them.

- Use the media: relevant journalists need to be engaged to ensure that research messages can be incorporated into the media's schedules.
- Use a combination of dissemination methods such as newsletters; websites; linking with existing databases; use of different formats (such as audiotape, video and CD-ROM); use of print and broadcast media; research syntheses/reviews; involving local practitioners and policy-makers to spell out implications of research; targeted mailing of research summaries to policy-makers and practitioners; invitation seminars; appropriate summaries for service users and user involvement in planning dissemination.
- Be proactive by contacting agencies directly.
- Understand external factors such as political sensitivities, financial and administrative mechanisms.

The *Framework for Progam Evaluation in Public Health* (Milstein and Wetterhall 1999) suggests that 'Facilitating use of evaluation findings also carries with it the responsibility for preventing misuse'. Such misuse might include taking findings out of context, making inappropriate generalizations from a single study or overemphasizing positive or negative findings. The *Framework* encourages active follow-up of how the findings are being used to ensure that they are not misrepresented or falsely applied.

The wider picture

In this final section we will turn our attention to the issue of generalization of findings and their contribution to the evidence base. We noted in Chapter 3 the so-called efficacy paradox which refers to the assessment of outcomes of an intervention delivered under ideal circumstances, when its effectiveness in the less perfect world of everyday practice may not be known. Actual effectiveness in the field will be the product not only of the effect of a programme on the recipients themselves, but also of the proportion and characteristics of the population reached, the uptake and delivery of the programme and sustainability of change in either organizations or individuals. The RE-AIM framework has its origins in the concerns of Glasgow *et al.* (1999) about the emphasis on efficacy and internal validity in evaluations and limited transferability of findings to 'real' situations. The RE-AIM framework can be used as an evaluation tool, but it can also be applied to the assessment or reporting of evaluation findings to ensure that key variables concerning wider transferability are addressed. It provides essential information to inform decisions about the programme, including acceptability to organizations and staff. The framework (see RE-AIM 2004) includes five dimensions:

Reach – the absolute number, proportion, and representiveness of individuals who participate in a programme.
Efficacy/effectiveness – includes the achievement of important outcomes, quality of life and costs and also any potential negative effects.

Adoption – the absolute number, proportion, and representativeness of settings and staff who are willing to use the programme.

Implementation – the faithfulness with which staff implement the programme, including consistency of delivery and the time and cost of the programme.

Maintenance – the extent to which a programme or policy becomes part of routine practices. This can also apply to the maintenance of change at the individual level among those targeted by the programme.

In recent years there has been increasing emphasis on using evidence to guide practice within health promotion and public health. The cornerstone of evidence-based practice is generally held to be empirical research and evaluation, as reflected in the following definitions:

> an approach that incorporates into policy and practice decision processes the findings from a critical evaluation of demonstrated evaluation effects.
> (Rychetnik and Wise 2004: 248)

> the systematic integration of research evidence into the planning and implementation of health promotion activities.
> (Wiggers and Sanson-Fisher 1998: 141)

This emphasis on the use of evaluation findings has fuelled attempts to appraise and synthesize evidence. However, there are concerns that there is a mismatch between the evidence available and both the current health agenda and the needs of practitioners. Firstly, the existing evaluation evidence is dominated by simple interventions focusing on changing individual or small-group behaviour rather than tackling the more complex 'upstream' determinants of health and health action (Rychetnik and Wise 2004). Secondly, interventions tend to focus on a small range of risk behaviours. For example, Oldenburg *et al.*'s (1999) audit found that 76 per cent of papers on health promotion research were concerned with behaviours associated with cardiovascular disease and cancer, in contrast to only 1 per cent on mental health. Thirdly, programme failures are rarely reported, yet there is potentially much to be learned from an analysis of what went wrong and why. Fourthly, published reviews are primarily concerned with outcomes rather than identifying the processes or contextual factors associated with the achievement of outcomes. Barry *et al.* (2005: 30) note that 'As a result there is a dearth of published information to guide practitioners and decision-makers regarding the practical aspects of programme adoption and replication'.

Notwithstanding the emphasis on evidence, professional expertise and practitioner experience are also recognized as being important (Sackett *et al.* 1996). This point was recognized by the Health Development Agency in England in developing its strategy for getting evidence into practice in public health:

> To determine whether an intervention, even one well founded in evidence, is likely to be successful requires an understanding of local contexts and circumstances, of local professionals' knowledge bases, commitment and

engagement, and detailed assessment of the population at whom the intervention is aimed. (Kelly *et al*. 2004b: 5)

As well as producing 'evidence briefings' which synthesize review-level evidence, the HDA developed an approach for involving practitioners in assessing the relevance of findings to practice. These are published as 'effective action briefings' (Kelly *et al*. 2004b).

There continues to be controversy about the different value afforded to different types of research in the selection of evaluations for inclusion in systematic reviews – the hierarchy being headed by the randomized controlled trial (see, for example, Perkins *et al*. 1999; Kelly *et al*. 2002). It is not appropriate to revisit that debate here. Suffice it to say that there is growing support for the use of a wider range of evidence and the development of approaches for integrating qualitative and quantitative evidence (see, for example, Dixon-Woods *et al*. 2004, 2005).

There are concerns that empirical evidence alone is insufficient to direct practice and that we need to draw out the general principles that would inform wider application. The development of theory can enhance understanding of complex situations and the interactions within them (Green 2000). Although practitioners are often sceptical about the value of theory, Buchanan (1994: 274) takes the view that this is due to a narrow view of theory and proposes a broader conceptualization which recognizes that 'knowledge is contingent and contextual rather than universal, determinate and invariable'. The development of theory then, can incorporate contextual factors and practitioner and community insights and has both explanatory and predictive capability, that is, it sheds light on what has happened and gives practitioners some idea of what might happen if they were to attempt to replicate the intervention in a different context. Using evaluation findings to develop or refine theory can produce general principles to inform practice.

Pawson (2002) is concerned that the emphasis of traditional systematic reviews of evidence is on the potential contribution of interventions to achieving some broad health outcome, such as injury prevention or reduction in teenage pregnancy. Further, the 'same yardstick' tends to be applied to completely dissimilar interventions (see Box 9.4). He contends that it is not programmes that work, but it is the resources a programme brings that allow subjects to generate change. The extent to which change is 'triggered' will be heavily influenced by the context. It is therefore false logic to assume that programmes can be judged as effective or not without due reference to the characteristics of the target group and context. He proposes that a realist synthesis of evidence offers a 'transferable theory' about what works for whom and in what circumstances. Its orientation is towards generative themes and their applicability in different situations rather than simple cause–effect relationships. So, for example, consideration could be given to the use of incentives or 'giveaways', such as smoke alarms, to identify in what contexts, for which groups and for what purposes this type of approach may or may not work.

Box 9.4 Different approaches to injury prevention

1. Free smoke alarms

Intended mechanism:

Make a resource available.

Subjects can be persuaded to accept, install, maintain and act on the alarm sounding.

2. School road safety education

Intended mechanism:

Passing on codes about behaviour in traffic.

Children will be able to recall and apply the rules in a specific road situation.

Points for reflection

What would you expect to see in an evaluation report to enable you to understand the context and mechanism for each?

Summary

Clearly, if evaluation is to fulfil its purpose of informing policy and practice, the findings need to be fed back to key stakeholder groups, both internal and external to the programme being evaluated. Understanding the needs of these various groups is fundamental to ensuring that evaluation reports include relevant information, communicate it in an accessible way and are disseminated through appropriate channels. We have emphasized throughout this text that evaluation should include consideration of process and context, as well as outcomes, and address the complex interrelationships between them. Notwithstanding preferences among stakeholder groups for qualitative or qualitative evidence, deriving from differing epistemological positions, there is growing acceptance of the need to combine both perspectives in constructing the evidence base for public health. The quality of the evidence will ultimately depend on those involved in evaluation getting their findings into the public domain and including sufficient information to inform policy and practice decisions.

10 Conclusion

In this book we have looked at evaluation as one of the key concepts for public health practice. The principles underpinning evaluation, the core elements of practice and common dilemmas have all been examined in depth. We have tried to chart a pathway through the broad field of evaluation and illuminate some of the choices available to those working in public health and health promotion. We hope that our exploration of major influences on evaluation practice and the identification of a wide range of approaches are of use not only to those directly involved in the generation of evidence but also to commissioners and consumers of evaluation.

Evaluation needs to be an integral part of programme planning and development in order to answer the questions 'what works?' and 'why?'. Evaluation can be described as a systematic process for the purpose of producing evidence to inform decision-making and policy. We recognize that this essentially rationalist approach may sit uncomfortably in our post-modern age, but our contention is that the best evaluation is **structured**, **systematic**, **planned** and **reflective**. Lewis (2001) highlights the significance of evaluation for **learning** about programme effects and processes. This is compared to types of 'pseudo' evaluation (Suchman 1967, cited in Newburn 2001):

- Eyewash – focus on surface experiences
- Whitewash – covering up programme failure
- Submarine – political use of evaluation to undermine a programme
- Posture – ritual use of evaluation with no intent to use findings
- Postponement – evaluation undertaken to avoid or postpone action.

A framework, such as presented in Chapter 4, can assist in evaluation planning and aid the collection, interpretation and appraisal of evidence. Quality issues need to be addressed, but this does not mean evaluation should aspire to use a standard form, nor should designs always be measured against a 'gold standard', whether that gold standard is a randomized controlled trial or a participatory approach. As discussed earlier, a commitment to evidence-based practice means that evaluation is required to assess effectiveness and, at the same time, ethical principles relating to both research and professional practice should be upheld. Chapter 2 identified the need for evaluation to be pragmatic and appropriate for purpose. We offer ten practical tips for commissioners and evaluators in Boxes 10.1 and 10.2 at the end of this final chapter.

Many of the issues discussed in the book relating to the design and conduct of evaluation are applicable to different types of programmes, from small projects to large regional or national initiatives. They are also applicable to programmes both in health and non-health sectors. Indeed, in the current policy context, the assumption is that public health practitioners will require evaluation skills to operate in a number of sectors, not only health but also regeneration, education, community work, leisure and sport, to name but a few. There is undoubtedly some consistency about the broad principles of evaluation, nonetheless there remain some significant and distinct debates pertaining to evaluation within public health and health promotion. A number of themes have threaded through the book which link discussions on theory and praxis. Key issues discussed include:

- what counts as evidence in public health and health promotion
- measurement of health outcomes and selection of indicators
- the significance of process and context
- ensuring evaluation practice is equitable and inclusive
- the impact and value of collaboration and participation in the evaluation process.

Evidence and effectiveness remain contested concepts in public health and health promotion, yet in recent years the debates appear to have moved on. Somehow the notion that an allegiance to positivism or interpretivism is all that is required to inform decisions about evaluation misses the point. A paper from the Health Development Agency (Kelly *et al.* 2002) on some of the methodological problems in constructing the evidence base discusses the frustrations of having to traverse the 'fault line' between the two major epistemological positions. The paper goes on to argue:

> The problems of inequalities in mortality and morbidity, and finding appropriate interventions to reduce inequalities, are too pressing a task to deny the possibility of objectivism or subjectivism, if they might help. . . . in collating the evidence base for public health, we are faced with the challenge of developing an epistemological position that allows us to acknowledge a variety of intellectual and practical approaches to the nature of truths and reality, and turn these into something that is useful and applicable for practitioners in the field. (Kelly *et al.* 2002: 7)

We have reflected the pluralistic character of current evaluation theory and practice in the book. A good evaluator has a wealth of different approaches to draw on, all with their own underlying logic. We have favoured a realist approach as it provides a suitable framework for evaluation of complex initiatives. However, we acknowledge the value and utility of other approaches, from experimental to participatory.

Measurement issues have featured strongly in the book. While there has been a tendency in public health to focus on morbidity and mortality indicators, health promotion as a field has grappled with trying to devise valid indicators of health and well-being based on a social model of health. We have highlighted the challenges in defining good indicators for health.

Appropriate outcomes are often difficult to measure, particularly where they are concerned with fuzzy aspects such as empowerment. Changes in health status may be long-term, and there is a need for interim measures of effectiveness (Nutbeam 1998). Faced with the difficulty of measurement there are two tendencies. One is to abandon measurement but to maintain a conviction that what is being done is right. The alternative position is to count what appears countable, often limited to service outputs. Both positions, though caricatured here, are seen in practice. We have argued strongly that there are challenges in selecting and defining indicators, but also that it is possible to measure changes in people, in communities, in organizations and in populations. What is required is that outcomes, indicators of success and methods are linked and that indicators are selected on the basis that they are **valid** (that they measure what they set out to), **credible** (capable of convincing stakeholders) and **meaningful** (measurement will be correctly interpreted by stakeholders). Although a number of tools and resources have been highlighted throughout the book which can assist in defining indicators, there remains scope for development of different measures of success in health promotion and public health.

One aspect that we have returned to at different points is the need for evaluation to be contextualized. The settings for public health practice and the nature of target populations need to be taken in account in undertaking evaluation. Decisions are not only made on the basis of pragmatism, considering only what would or could work, but should also be informed by the values and principles of practice. Whatever research approach is adopted, we have argued that evaluation has to fit with the ethos of programmes. Furthermore, public health evaluation should support aims around the pursuit of equity and not undermine attempts to reduce health inequalities. Such aspirations place heavy responsibilities on evaluators and there are likely to be genuine difficulties faced in real-life situations, especially where groups are hard to reach. Expectations about what is considered 'proper' research can have the effect of undermining the confidence of evaluators to address the challenges found in practice.

Another theme has been the importance of collaboration. Research rarely conforms to the stereotypical model of individual, independent study and certainly evaluation is by its nature a collaborative activity. Evaluation is integral to the development of a well-planned programme and therefore there has to be involvement from those developing, managing and implementing the programme, as well as from the participants and beneficiaries. The extensive literature around collaborative and participatory evaluation points to the benefits of seeking wider stakeholder involvement in planning and undertaking evaluation and in dissemination. We have set out the justifications for participation in the evaluation process, different types of approaches to consider and some of the pitfalls. Choices over the extent and level of participation will vary with the context, but we recommend that the best evaluations are based on the principles of partnership working. Wide ownership of evaluation can lead to better learning in programmes.

Finally, the book has touched on many different strategies, methods, designs, measures and resources for evaluation. The diversity of approaches is perhaps to be expected given the diversity within public health and health promotion practice. We all need a range of options in order to undertake robust evaluation in different contexts. Given the challenges for practice-based evaluation, dogma about methodologies and methods seems out of place and unnecessarily limiting. At each stage of the evaluation journey we need to consider, select and appraise available options. Choices should be justified against the drive for evidence, programme goals, situational and contextual factors, and the needs of the stakeholders. Reflection and critical analysis are part of that process. We have tried to put forward some practical, grounded strategies which can be adapted for evaluation in different settings. We hope that those engaged in evaluation will feel confident to use and adapt these strategies and take up opportunities to enable different voices to be heard. Evaluators do not always get things right and therefore there needs to be transparency about the selection of methods and the reality of implementation. We hope that overall this book has given readers the knowledge and tools to make valid choices about evaluation in practice.

Box 10.1 Ten tips for evaluators

1 Draw up an evaluation plan at the beginning of the evaluation process.
2 Identify relevant indicators of success and use them to guide the selection of methods and collection of data; but also remain open to unanticipated outcomes.
3 Examine process and context as well as outcome; explanations about how and why a programme works are useful.
4 Design and methods should fit with the values and ethos of the programme.
5 Seek stakeholder involvement to enhance the relevance and utility of the evaluation.
6 Use different perspectives and multiple methods to strengthen the evidence.
7 Ethical issues need to be considered throughout the evaluation.
8 Be prepared to use innovative solutions to overcome barriers and problems.
9 Ensure that the main findings are clearly presented and accessible to different audiences.
10 Be honest about the evidence and its limitations.

Box 10.2 Ten tips for commissioners of evaluation

1 Ensure sufficient resources are devoted to evaluation to allow useful evidence to be collected.

2 Make sure that programme goals, objectives and underpinning values are clearly articulated and understood by those involved in evaluation.

3 Address the issue of evaluation at the planning stage of an intervention, not at the end.

4. Make your expectations clear, define the scope of the evaluation, agree an evaluation plan, and allocate responsibilities.

5 Seek to encourage and facilitate wider stakeholder involvement in the evaluation.

6 Provide a clear steer and support for staff engaging in participatory evaluation.

7 Maintain a dialogue with evaluators throughout a project.

8 Be open to new ideas and approaches which may lead to innovation and improved evaluation practice.

9 Allocate adequate time and resources to dissemination; do not let the final report sit on the shelf.

10 Learn from the evidence and use the findings.

References

ActKnowledge and Aspen Institute Roundtable on Community Change (n.d.) *Theory of Change: Overview.* http://www.theoryofchange.org/html/overview.html (accessed 1 March 2006).

Allan, D. (2004) *The National Evaluation of the Children's Fund: Some Recommendations for the Commissioning and Use of Local Evaluation.* NECF. http://www.ne-cf.org/core_files/lets%20final%20draft%202.doc (accessed 1 March 2006).

Allan, D., Barnes, M., Coad, J., Fielding, A., Hansen, K., Mathers, J., McCabe, A., Morris, K., Parry, J., Plewis, I., Prior, D. and Sullivan, A. (2004) *Assessing the Impact of the Children's Fund: The Role of Indicators.* National Evaluation of the Children's Fund. http://www.ne-cf.org/core_files/CF%20indicators%20paper%20final.doc (accessed 1 March 2006).

Allison, K. and Rootman, I. (1996) Scientific rigor and community participation in health promotion research: are they compatible? *Health Promotion International,* 11(4): 333–40.

Alsop, R. and Heinsohn, N. (2005) *Measuring Empowerment in Practice: Structuring Analysis and Framing Indicators.* World Bank Policy Research Working Paper 3510, http://econ.worldbank.org/files/41307_wps3510.pdf (accessed 1 March 2006).

American Evaluation Association (2004) *Guiding Principles for Evaluators.* http://www.eval.org/Publications/GuidingPrinciples.asp (accessed 23 January 2006).

Anyanwu, C.N. (1988) The technique of participatory research in community development, *Community Development Journal,* 23(1): 11–15.

Ashdown, J. (n.d.) *A Story to Be Told.* London: Barnardo's.

Aspen Institute (n.d.) *Theory of Change Origins.* http://www.theoryofchange.org/html/origins.html (accessed 7 September 2005).

Autier, P., Doré, J., Négrier, S., Liénard, D., Panizzon, R., Lejeune, F.J., Guggisberg, D. and Eggermont, A.M.M. (1999) Sunscreen use and duration of sun exposure: a double-blind, randomized trial, *Journal of the National Cancer Institute,* 91(15): 1304–9.

Backett-Milburn, K. and McKie, L. (1999) A critical appraisal of the draw and write technique, *Health Education Research,* 14(3): 387–98.

Banks, S. (2003) The concept of 'community practice', in S. Banks, H. Butcher, P. Henderson and J. Robertson (eds) *Managing Community Practice. Principles, Policies, and Programmes.* Bristol: Policy Press.

Barlow, J., Kirkpatrick, S., Stewart-Brown, S. and Davis, H. (2005) Hard-to-reach or out-of-reach? Reasons why women refuse to take part in early interventions, *Children and Society,* 19: 199–210.

Barnardo's Research and Development Team (2000) *Linking Research and Practice.* Joseph Rowntree Foundation Findings Report. http://www.jrf.org.uk/knowledge/findings/socialcare/910.asp (accessed 1 March 2006).

Barnes, M. (1999) Researching public participation, *Local Government Studies,* 25(4): 60–75.

Barnes, M., Matka, E. and Sullivan, H. (2003) Evidence, understanding and complexity, *Evaluation,* 9(3): 265–84.

Barr, A. (2003) Participative planning and evaluation skills, in S. Banks, H. Butcher, P. Henderson and J. Robertson (eds) *Managing Community Practice. Principles, Policies, and Programmes*. Bristol: Policy Press.

Barr, A. and Hashagen, S. (2000) *ABCD Handbook. A Framework for Evaluating Community Development*. London: Community Development Foundation.

Barr, A., Hashagen, S. and Purcell, R. (1996) *Measuring Community Development in Northern Ireland: A Handbook for Practitioners*. Belfast: Voluntary Activity Unit, Department of Health and Social Services (Northern Ireland).

Barreto, M.L. (2005) Efficacy, effectiveness, and the evaluation of public health interventions, *Journal of Epidemiology and Community Health*, 59: 345–6.

Barry, M.B., Domitrovich, C. and Lara, A. (2005) The implementation of mental health programmes, *Promotion & Education*, Special Edition, 2: 30–5.

Basch, P.F. and Gold, R.S. (1986) The dubious effects of type V errors in hypothesis testing on health education practice and theory, *Health Education Research*, 1(4): 299–305.

Baum, F. (1995) Researching public health: beyond the qualitative–quantitative methodological debate, *Social Science and Medicine*, 40(4): 459–68.

Baum, F. (1998) Measuring effectiveness in community-based health promotion, in J.K. Davies and G. MacDonald (eds) *Quality, Evidence and Effectiveness in Health Promotion. Striving for Certainties*. London: Routledge.

Beattie, A. (1995) Evaluation in community development for health: an opportunity for dialogue, *Health Education Journal*, 54: 465–72.

Benoit, C., Jansson, M., Millar, A. and Phillips, R. (2005) Community-academic research on hard-to-reach populations: benefits and challenges, *Qualitative Health Research*, 15(2): 263–82.

Beresford, P. (2003) User involvement in research: exploring the challenges, *NT Research*, 8(1): 36–46.

Bhopal, R., Vettini, A., Hunt, S., *et al.* (2004) Review of prevalence data in, and evaluation of methods for cross cultural adaptation of, UK surveys on tobacco and alcohol in ethnic minority groups, *British Medical Journal*, 328: 76–80.

Biott, C. and Cook, T. (2000) Local evaluation in a National Early Years Excellence Centres Pilot Programme, *Evaluation*, 6(4): 399–413.

Bjärås, G., Haglund, B.J.A. and Rifkin, S.B. (1991) A new approach to community participation assessment, *Health Promotion International*, 6(3): 199–206.

Black, D. (1998) The limitations of evidence, *Journal of the Royal College of Physicians of London*, 32(1): 23–6.

Blenkinsop, S., Eggers, M., Schagen, I., Schagen, S., Scott, E., Warwick, I., Aggleton, P., Chase, E., with Zuurmond, M.A. (2004) *Evaluation of the Impact of the National Healthy School Standard: Final Report*, Thomas Coran Research Unit and National Foundation for Educational Research. http://www.wiredforhealth.gov.uk/PDF/Full_report_2004.pdf (accessed 8 September 2005).

Bodart, C. and Sapirie, S. (1998) Defining essential information needs and indicators, *World Health Forum*, 19: 303–9.

BOND (n.d.) *Monitoring and Evaluation*, Guidance Notes No. 4.3. London: BOND. www.bond.org.uk/pubs/guidance/4monitorandevaluate.pdf (accessed 7 September 2005).

Bonnell, C. (2002) The utility of randomised controlled trials of social interventions: an examination of two trials of HIV prevention, *Critical Public Health*, 12(4): 321–34.

Bonner, L. (2003) Using theory-based evaluation to build evidence-based health and social care policy and practice, *Critical Public Health*, 13(1): 77–92.

Boote, J., Telford, R. and Cooper, C. (2002) Consumer involvement in health research: a review and research agenda, *Health Policy*, 61: 213–36.

Boutilier, M., Mason, R. and Rootman, I. (1997) Community action and reflective practice in health promotion research, *Health Promotion International*, 12(1): 69–78.

Bowling, A. (1997a) *Measuring Health: A Review of Quality of Life Measurement Scales*, 2nd edn. Buckingham: Open University Press.

Bowling, A. (1997b) *Research Methods in Health*. Buckingham: Open University Press.

Boyd, P. (2003) Health research and the Data Protection Act 1998, *Journal of Health Services Research and Policy*, 8 (Suppl. 1): 24–7.

British Psychological Society (2004) *Ethical Principles for Conducting Research with Human Participants*. http://www.bps.org.uk/the-society/ethics-rules-charter-code-of-conduct/code-of-conduct/ethical-principles-for-conducting-research-with-human-participants.cfm (accessed 19 July 2005).

Brodie, I. (2003) *The Involvement of Parents and Carers in Sure Start Local Evaluations*. National Evaluation of Sure Start. http://www.ness.bbk.ac.uk/documents/GuidanceReports/171.pdf (accessed 14 March 2006).

Brook, R. and Lohr, K. (1985) Efficiency, effectiveness, variations and quality, *Medical Care*, 23(5): 710–22.

Buchanan, D.R. (1994) Reflections on the relationship between theory and practice, *Health Education Research*, 9(3): 273–83.

Burns, D. and Taylor, M. (2000) *Auditing Community Participation*. Bristol: Policy Press, in association with the Joseph Rowntree Foundation.

Burrows, R., Bunton, R., Muncer, S. and Gillen, K. (1995) The efficacy of health promotion, health economics and late modernism, *Health Education Research*, 10(2): 241–9.

Burton, P., Croft, J., Hastings, A., *et al.* (2004) *What Works in Area-Based Initiatives? A Systematic Review of the Literature*. Home Office Online Report 53/04. http://www.active-citizen.org.uk/research_reports_details.asp?id=2004102211137&cat=7&parentid= (accessed 21 January 2006).

Butcher, H. (1993) Introduction: some examples and definitions, in H. Butcher, A. Glen, P. Henderson and G. Smith (eds) *Community and Public Policy*. London: Pluto Press.

Byford, S., McDaid, D. and Sefton, T. (2003) *Because It's Worth It – A Practical Guide to Conducting Economic Evaluations in the Social Welfare Field*. Joseph Rowntree Foundation. www.jrf.org.uk/bookshop/eBooks/1859351123.pdf (accessed 19 September 2005).

Campbell, M., Fitzpatrick, R., Haines, A., *et al.* (2000) Framework for design and evaluation of complex interventions to improve health, *British Medical Journal*, 321: 694–6.

Canadian Evaluation Society (n.d.) *The Program Evaluation Standards*. http://www.wmich.edu/evalctr/jc/PGMSTNDS-SUM.htm (accessed 23 January 2006).

Carr-Hill, R. and Chalmers Dixon, P. (2002) *A Review of Methods for Monitoring and Measuring Social Inequality, Deprivation and Health Inequality*. South East Public Health Observatory. http://www.ihs.ox.ac.uk/sepho/publications/carrhill/ (accessed 1 August 2002).

Carstairs, V. (1995) Deprivation indices: their interpretation and use in relation to health, *Journal of Epidemiology and Community Health*, 49 (Suppl. 2): S3–S8.

Celnick, A. (2000) Ethics in the field, in D. Burton (ed.) *Research Training for Social Scientists*. London: Sage.

Centers for Disease Control and Prevention (2003) *WISEWOMAN Works Vol. 1: A Collection of Success Stories from Program Inception through 2002*. Centers for Disease

Control and Prevention, National Center for Chronic Disease Prevention and Health Promotion. http://www.cdc.gov/wisewoman/ (accessed 5 December 2005).

Centers for Disease Control and Prevention (2005) *WISEWOMAN Works Vol. 2: A Collection of Success Stories on Empowering Women to Stop Smoking*. Centers for Disease Control and Prevention. http://www.cdc.gov/wisewoman/ (accessed 5 December 2005).

Central Office for Research Ethics Committees (n.d.) *About Us*. http://www.corec.org.uk/public/about/about.htm (accessed 23 January 2006).

Charlton, B.G. (1991) Medical practice and the double-blind randomised controlled trial, *British Journal of General Practice*, 42(350): 355–6.

Chen, H.-T. (1990) *Theory Driven Evaluation*. Newbury Park, CA: Sage.

Chief Medical Officer (2001) *The Report of the Chief Medical Officer's Project to Strengthen the Public Health Function*. London: Department of Health.

Clegg, M. (2002) *Commissioning evaluation: is there an enlightened approach?* UK Evaluation Society. www.evaluation.org.uk/conference/Conf%20presentations%202002/Clegg.pdf (accessed 13 July 2005).

Coad, J. and Lewis, A. (2004) *Engaging Children and Young People in Research. Literature review for the National Evaluation of the Children's Fund (NECF)*. Birmingham: National Evaluation of the Children's Fund. http://www.ne-cf.org/briefing.asp?section=000100040009&profile=000100080003 (accessed 22 January 2006).

Cohen, L. and Manion, L. (1994) *Research Methods in Education*, 4th edn. London: Routledge.

COMMIT Research Group (1991) Community Intervention Trial for Smoking Cessation (COMMIT): Summary of design and intervention, *Journal of the National Cancer Institute*, 83(22): 1620–8.

COMMIT Research Group (1995) Community Intervention Trial for Smoking Cessation (COMMIT): I. Cohort results from a four-year community intervention, *American Journal of Public Health*, 85(2): 183–92.

Community Development and Health Network (n.d.) *A Rough Guide to Learning for Healthy Communities through Evaluation*. http://www.cdhn.org/publications/index.asp (accessed 21 January 2006).

Connell, J.P. and Kubisch, A.C. (1998) Applying a theory of change approach to the evaluation of comprehensive community initiatives: progress, prospects, and problems, in K. Fulbright-Anderson, A.C. Kubisch, and J.P. Connell, *New Approaches to Evaluating Community Initiatives, Vol. 2: Theory, Measurement and Analysis*. Washington DC: Aspen Institute. http://www.aspeninstitute.org/site/c.huLWJeMRKpH/b.613709/k.B547/Applying_a_Theory_of_Change_Approach_to_the_Evaluation_of_Comprehensive_Community_Initiatives_Progress_Prospects_and_Problems.htm (accessed 15 August 2005).

Connelly, J. (2001) Critical realism and health promotion: effective practice needs an effective theory, *Health Education Research*, 16(2): 115–19.

Coombes, Y. (2000) Combining quantitative and qualitative approaches to evaluation, in M. Thorogood and Y. Coombes (eds) *Evaluating Health Promotion Practice and Methods*. Oxford: Oxford University Press.

Cornwall, A. and Jewkes, R. (1995) What is participatory research? *Social Science and Medicine*, 41(12): 1667–76.

Cote, S. and Healy, T. (2001) *The Well-being of Nations. The Role of Human and Social Capital*. Paris: Organisation for Economic Co-operation and Development.

Cotterill, L. (2002) Developing capacity for theory-based evaluation, in L. Bauld and K. Judge (eds) *Learning from Health Action Zones*. Chichester: Aeneas Press.

Craig, N. and Walker, D. (1996) Choice and accountability in health promotion: the role of health economics, *Health Education Research*, 11(3): 355–60.

Croft, S. and Beresford, P. (1992) The politics of participation, *Critical Social Policy*, 35: 20–43.

Crow, I. (2000) The power of research, in D. Burton (ed.) *Research Training for Social Scientists*. London: Sage.

Curtis, K., Roberts, H., Copperman, J., Downie, A. and Liabo, K. (2004) 'How come I don't get asked no questions?' Researching 'hard to reach' children and teenagers, *Child and Family Social Work*, 9: 167–75.

Daniel, P. and Dearden, P.N. (2001) *Integrating a Logical Framework Approach to Planning into the Health Action Zone Initiative*. HAZNET. http://www.haznet.org.uk/resources/ book_logical-framework.doc (accessed 22 May 2002).

Davey Smith, G., Ebrahim, S. and Frankel, S. (2005) How policy informs the evidence, *British Medical Journal*, 322(7280): 184–5.

Davies, H., Nutley, S. and Tilley, N. (2000) Debates on the role of experimentation, in H. Davies, S. Nutley and P. Smith (eds) *What Works? Evidence Based Policy and Practice*. Bristol: Policy Press.

De Koning, K. and Martin, M. (eds) (1996) *Participatory Research in Health. Issues and Experiences*. London: Zed Books.

Denzin, N.K. (1970) *The Research Act in Sociology*. London: Butterworths.

Department of Health (1998) *Chief Medical Officer's Report to Strengthen the Public Health Function in England*. London: HMSO.

Department of Health (1999) *Saving Lives: Our Healthier Nation*, Cm 4386. London: Stationery Office.

Department of Health (2001a) *Research Governance Framework for Health and Social Care*. London: Department of Health.

Department of Health (2001b) *Shifting the Balance of Power within the NHS: Securing Delivery*. http://www.dh.gov.uk/assetRoot/04/07/65/22/04076522.pdf (accessed 6 March 2006).

Department of Health (2005a) *Choosing Health: Planning and Performance Toolkit for PCTs and their Partners*. Department of Health. http://www.bashh.org/ committees/cgc/choosing_health_wp_pcy_toolkit210205.doc (accessed 30 September 2005).

Department of Health (2005b) *Research Governance Framework for Health and Social Care*, 2nd edn. Department of Health. http://www.dh.gov.uk/assetRoot/04/12/24/27/ 04122427.pdf (accessed 15 March 2006).

Department of Health (2005c) *Tackling Health Inequalities: Status Report on the Programme for Action*. Department of Health. http://www.dh.gov.uk/assetRoot/04/ 11/76/98/04117698.pdf (accessed 15 March 2006).

Department of Human Services (2005) *Evaluation and Dissemination*. Department of Human Services, State Government of Victoria. http://www.health.vic.gov.au/ healthpromotion/hp_practice/eval_dissem.htm#narrative (accessed 24 October 2005).

Dibben, C., Sims, A., Watson, J., Barnes, H., Smith, T., Sigala, M., Hill, A. and Manley, D. (2004) *Health Poverty Index Visualisation Tool*. South East Public Health Observatory, Oxford. http://www.hpi.org.uk/indicators.php (accessed 30 October 2005).

Dickson, G. and Green, K.L. (2001) Participatory action research: lessons learned with Aboriginal grandmothers, *Health Care for Women International*, 22: 471–82.

Dixon, J. (1995) Community stories and indicators for evaluating community development, *Community Development Journal*, 30(4): 327–36.

Dixon-Woods, M., Agarwal, S., Young, B., Jones, D. and Sutton, A. (2004) *Integrative*

Approaches to Qualitative and Quantitative Evidence. London: Health Development Agency.

Dixon-Woods, M., Agarwal, S., Jones, D., Young, B. and Sutton, A. (2005) Synthesising qualitative and quantitative evidence: a review of possible methods, *Journal of Health Services Research and Policy*, 10(1): 45–53.

Eakin, J., Robertson, A., Poland, B., Coburn, D. and Edwards, R. (1996) Towards a critical social science perspective on health promotion research, *Health Promotion International*, 11(2): 157–65.

Eby, M. (2000) Producing evidence ethically, in R. Gomm and C. Davies (eds) *Using Evidence in Health and Social Care*. London: Sage.

Edgar, A., Salek, S., Shickle, D. and Cohen, D. (1998) *The Ethical QALY: Ethical Issues in Healthcare Resource Allocations*. Haslemere: Euromed Communications Ltd.

Editor *BMJ* (1998) Fifty years of randomised controlled trials. *British Medical Journal*, 317(7167). http://bmj.bmjjournals.com/cgi/content/full/317/7167/0 (accessed 2 March 2006).

Edwards, S.J.L., Lilford, R.J. and Hewison, J. (1998) The ethics of randomised controlled trials from the perspective of patients, the public and healthcare professionals, *British Medical Journal*, 317: 1209–12.

Edwards, S.J.L., Braunholtz, D.A., Lilford, R.J. and Stevens, A.J. (1999) Ethical issues in the design and conduct of cluster randomised controlled trials, *British Medical Journal*, 318: 1407–9.

Effective Interventions Unit (2002) *Evaluation Guide 8. Evaluating Outreach Services.* http://www.drugmisuse.isdscotland.org/goodpractice/EIU_evaluationg8.pdf (accessed 10 November 2005).

El Ansari, W.E., Phillips, C.J. and Hammick, M. (2001) Collaboration and partnerships: developing the evidence base, *Health and Social Care in the Community*, 9(4): 215–27.

Elliston, K.M. (2002) Establishing a 'code of ethical research practice' in health promotion – a discussion paper, *International Journal of Health Promotion and Education*, 40(1): 15–20.

Entwistle, V., Renfrew, M.J., Yearley, J., Forrester, J. and Lamont, T. (1998) Lay perspectives: advantages for health research, *British Medical Journal*, 316: 463–6.

Euroqol (n.d.) *EQ–5D.* Euroqol Group http://www.euroqol.org/content.htm (accessed 19 March 2002).

Fairfax, P., Green, E., Hawran, H., South, J. and Cairns, L. (2002) *Well Connected! A Self Assessment Tool on Community Involvement for Organisations.* Bradford: Bradford Metropolitan District Council, Bradford Health Action Zone.

Fawcett, S.B., Paine-Andrews, A., Francisco, V.T., *et al.* (2001) Evaluating community health initiatives for health and development, in I. Rootman, M.S. Goodstadt, B. Hyndman, D.V. McQueen, L. Potvin, J. Springett and E. Ziglio (eds) *Evaluation in Health Promotion. Principles and Perspectives*. Copenhagen: WHO Europe.

Fetterman, D. (n.d.) *Empowerment Evaluation: Collaboration, Action Research, and a Case Example.* Action Evaluation Research Institute. http://www.aepro.org/inprint/ conference/fetterman.html (accessed 29 October 2005).

Fetterman, D. and Wandersman, A. (2005) *Empowerment Evaluation Principles in Practice.* New York: Guilford Publications.

Feuerstein, M.T. (1986) *Partners in Evaluation. Evaluating Development and Community Programmes with Participants.* London: Macmillan.

Fisher, R.A. (1949) *The Design of Experiments*, 5th edn. Edinburgh: Oliver & Boyd.

Fulbright-Anderson, K., Kubisch, A.C. and Connell, J.P. (eds) (1998) *New Approaches to Evaluating Community Initiatives, Vol. 2: Theory, Measurement and Analysis.* Washington DC: Aspen Institute. http://www.aspeninstitute.org/site/

c.huLWJeMRKpH/b.613721/k.17D2/New_Approaches_to_Evaluating_Community_Initiatives_Vol_2_Theory_Measurement_and_Analysis.htm (accessed 16 August 2005).

Funnell, R., Oldfield, K. and Speller, V. (1995) *Towards Healthier Alliances: A Tool for Planning, Evaluating and Developing Healthy Alliances*. London: Health Education Authority, Wessex Institute for Health.

Gabbay, M. and Gabby, J. (1997) Assessing the needs of hard-to-reach groups, in A. Harris (ed.) *Needs to Know? A Guide to Needs Assessment for Primary Care*. Edinburgh: Churchill Livingston.

Gallagher, B., Creighton, S. and Gibbons, J. (1995) Ethical dilemmas in social research: no easy solutions, *British Journal of Social Work*, 25: 295–311.

Gillam, S. and Levenson, R. (1999) Linkworkers in primary care, *British Medical Journal*, 319: 1215.

Glasgow, R.E., Vogt, T.M. and Boles, S.M. (1999) Evaluating the public health impact of health promotion interventions: The RE-AIM framework, *American Journal of Public Health*, 89: 1323–7.

Goddard, M. and Smith, P. (2001) Equity of access to health care services: theory and evidence from the UK, *Social Science and Medicine*, 53: 1149–62.

Godfrey, C. (2001) Economic evaluation of health promotion, in I. Rootman, M. Goodstadt, B. Hyndman, D.V. McQueen, L. Potvin, J. Springett and E. Ziglio (eds) *Evaluation in Health Promotion: Principles and Perspectives*. Copenhagen: WHO Europe.

Gomm, R., Needham, G. and Bullman, A. (2000) *Evaluating Research*. London: Sage.

Goodstadt, M.S., Hyndman, B., McQueen, D.V., Potvin, L., Rootman, I. and Springett, J. (2001) Evaluation in health promotion: synthesis and recommendations, in I. Rootman, M.S. Goodstadt, B. Hyndman, D.V. McQueen, L. Potvin, J. Springett and E. Ziglio (eds) *Evaluation in Health Promotion. Principles and Perspectives*. Copenhagen: WHO Europe.

Granger, R.C. (1998) Establishing causality in evaluations of comprehensive community initiatives, in K. Fulbright-Anderson, A.C. Kubisch and J.P. Connell (eds) *New Approaches to Evaluating Community Initiatives, Vol.2: Theory, Measurement and Analysis*. Washington, DC: Aspen Institute. http://www.aspeninstitute.org/site/c.huLWJeMRKpH/b.613721/k.17D2/New_Approaches_to_Evaluating_Community_Initiatives_Vol_2_Theory_Measurement_and_Analysis.htm (accessed 7 September 2005).

Green, J. (2000) Editorial: The role of theory in evidence-based health promotion practice, *Health Education Research*, 15(2): 125–9.

Green, J. and Camidge, D. (2001) *Evaluation of the UK Launch of the SMARTRISK Heroes Programme*. Leeds: Centre for Health Promotion Research, Leeds Metropolitan University.

Green, J. and Newell, C. (2003) *Evaluation of the Bingley Young People's Health Project*. Leeds: Centre for Health Promotion Research, Leeds Metropolitan University.

Green, J. and Tones, K. (1999) Towards a secure evidence base for health promotion, *Journal of Public Health Medicine*, 21(2): 133–9.

Green, L.W. (1977) Evaluation and measurement: some dilemmas for health education, *American Journal of Public Health*, 67(2): 155–61.

Green, L.W. and Richard, L. (1993) The need to combine health education and health promotion: the case of cardiovascular disease prevention, *Promotion & Education*, 0: 11–17.

Guardian (2005) Shaky times for Sure Start, *The Guardian*, 13 September.

Guba, E.G. and Lincoln, Y.S. (1989) *Fourth Generation Evaluation*. San Francisco: Jossey-Bass.

Gulliford, M., Figueroa-Munoz, J., Morgan, M., Hughes, D., Gibson, B., Beech, R. and Hudson, M. (2002) What does 'access to health care' mean? *Journal of Health Services Research and Policy*, 7(3): 186–8.

Hamer, M. and Box, V. (2000) An evaluation of the development and functioning of the Boscombe Network for Change, a health alliance or partnership for health in Dorset, *Health Education Journal*, 59: 238–52.

Handy, C. (1994) *The Empty Raincoat*. London: Hutchison.

Hanley, B., Truesdale, A., King, A., Elbourne, D. and Chalmers, I. (2001) Involving consumers in designing, conducting and interpreting randomised controlled trials: questionnaire survey, *British Medical Journal*, 322: 519–23.

Hanley, B., Bradburn, J., Barnes, M., *et al.* (2004) *Involving the Public in NHS Public Health and Social Care Research*, 2nd edn. Eastleigh: INVOLVE.

Haour-Knipe, M., Fleury, F. and Dubois-Arber, F. (1999) HIV/AIDS prevention for migrants and ethnic communities: three phases of evaluation, *Social Science and Medicine*, 49: 1357–72.

Harper, G.W. and Carver, L.J. (1999) 'Out-of-the-mainstream' youth as partners in collaborative research: exploring the benefits and challenges, *Health Education and Behavior*, 26(2): 250–65.

Harper, R. and Kelly, M. (2003) *Measuring Social Capital in the United Kingdom*. Office for National Statistics http://www.statistics.gov.uk/socialcapital/downloads/harmonisation_steve_5.pdf (accessed 2 March 2006).

Hart, E. and Bond, M. (1995) *Action Research for Health and Social Care. A Guide to Practice*. Buckingham: Open University Press.

Hashagen, S. (2003) Frameworks for measuring community health and well being, in J. Orme, J. Powell, P. Taylor, T. Harrison and M. Grey (eds) *Public Health for the 21st Century. New Perspectives on Policy, Participation and Practice*. Berkshire: Open University Press.

Hawe, P. (1994) Capturing the meaning of 'community' in community intervention evaluation: some contributions from community psychology, *Health Promotion International*, 9(3): 199–210.

Hawe, P., Shiell, A. and Riley, T. (2004) Complex interventions: how 'out of control' can a randomised controlled trial be? *British Medical Journal*, 328: 1561–3.

Hayes, M. and Manson Willms, S. (1990) Healthy community indicators: the perils of the search and the paucity of the find, *Health Promotion International*, 5(2): 161–6.

Health Communication Unit (2006) *Evaluating Health Promotion Programs Version 3.4.* Health Communication Unit, Centre for Health Promotion, University of Toronto. http://www.thcu.ca/infoandresources/evaluation_resources.htm (accessed 28 February 2006).

Health Development Agency (2002) *Case Studies of the Role of Health Promotion in Tackling Inequalities in Health, 1999–2000. European Network of Health Promotion Agencies UK National Report*. London: Health Development Agency.

Health Education Board for Scotland (HEBS) (n.d.) *HEBS Research & Evaluation Toolbox*. http://www.hebs.com/retoolbox/eval/hebsframe.html (accessed 21 January 2006).

Henderson, J., Torn, A. and Lucas, J. (2002) *Evaluation of Bradford Health Action Zone 1999–2002*. Bradford: University of Bradford.

Hepworth, J. (1997) Evaluation in health outcomes research: linking theories, methodologies and practice in health promotion, *Health Promotion International*, 12(3): 233–8.

Herman, J.L., Morris, L.L. and Fitz-Gibbon, C.T. (1987) *The Evaluator's Handbook*. Newbury Park, CA: Sage.

Holden, C. and Downie, A. (2002) Evaluating the evaluators: the role of evaluation in Health Action Zones: some lessons learnt, in L. Bauld and K. Judge (eds) *Learning from Health Action Zones*. Chichester: Aeneas Press.

Holman, B. (1987) Research from the underside, *British Journal of Social Work*, 17: 669–83.

Horrocks, C. and Blyth, E. (2003) Service user evaluations: young people, participation and client-centredness, *Youth and Policy*, 82(Winter): 16–26.

Hubley, J. (2002) *Health Empowerment, Health Literacy and Health Promotion – Putting It All Together – Working draft*. http://www.hubley.co.uk/1hlthempow.htm (accessed 29 October 2005).

Hughes, M. and Traynor, T. (2000) Reconciling process and outcome in evaluating community initiatives, *Evaluation*, 6(1): 37–49.

Hunt, S. (1987) Evaluating a community development project. Issues of acceptability, *British Journal of Social Work*, 17: 661–7.

Hurworth, R. (2004) The use of visual medium for program evaluation, *Studies in Qualitative Methodology*, 7(1): 163–81.

Information Commissioner (n.d.) *What Is the Data Protection Act (DPA)?* Data Protection Act Factsheet http://www.informationcommissioner.gov.uk/cms/DocumentUploads/Data%20Protection%20Act%20Fact%20V2.pdf (accessed 25 January 2006).

INVOLVE (2003) *A Guide to Paying Members of the Public Who Are Actively Involved in Research: For Researchers and Research Commissioners (Who May Also Be People Who Use Services)*. Eastleigh: INVOLVE.

Jackson, N. and Waters, E. (2005) Criteria for the systematic review of health promotion and public health interventions, *Health Promotion International*, 20(4): 367–74.

Jewkes, R. (2000) Evaluating community development initiatives in health promotion, in M. Thorogood and Y. Coombes (eds) *Evaluating Health Promotion Practice and Methods*. Oxford: Oxford University Press.

Johnson, J.L., Green, L.W., Frankish, C.J., MacLean, D.R. and Stachenko, S. (1996) A dissemination research agenda to strengthen health promotion and disease prevention, *Canadian Journal of Public Health*, 87(Suppl. 2): S5–S10.

Judd, J., Frankish, J. and Moulton, G. (2001) Setting standards in the evaluation of community based health promotion programmes – a unifying approach, *Health Promotion International*, 16(4): 367–80.

Judge, K. (2000) Testing evaluation to the limits: the case of English Health Action Zones. *Journal of Health Services Research and Policy*. http://www.haznet.org.uk/hazs/evidence/judge.asp (accessed 2 March 2006).

Judge, K. and Bauld, L. (2001) Strong theory, flexible methods: evaluating complex community-based initiatives, *Critical Public Health*, 11(1): 19–38.

Judge, K., Bauld, L., Barnes, M., *et al.* (1999) *Health Action Zones: Learning to Make a Difference. Findings from a Preliminary Review of Health Action Zones and Proposals for a National Evaluation. A Report Submitted to the Department of Health*. PSSRU Discussion Paper 1546. Canterbury: University of Kent.

Kaduskar, S., Boaz, A., Dowler, E., Meyrick, J. and Rayner, M. (1999) Evaluating the work of a community cafe in a town in the South East of England: reflections on methods, process, results, *Health Education Journal*, 58: 341–54.

Kane, R., Wellings, K., Free, C. and Goodrich, J. (2000) Uses of routine data sets in the evaluation of health promotion interventions: opportunities and limitations, *Health Education*, 100(1): 33–41.

Kaneko, M. (1999) A methodological inquiry into the evaluation of smoking cessation programmes, *Health Education Research*, 14(3): 433–41.

Katz, J. and Peberdy, A. (1997) *Promoting Health: Knowledge and Practice*. Basingstoke: Macmillan.

Kelly, M., Swann, C., Killoran, A., Naidoo, B., Barnett-Paige, E. and Morgan, A. (2002) *Methodological Problems in Constructing the Evidence Base in Public Health*. London: Health Development Agency. http://www.publichealth.nice.org.uk/ page.aspx?o=508135 (accessed 22 January 2006).

Kelly, M.P., Chambers, J., Huntley, J. and Millward, L. (2004a) *Method 1 for the Production of Effective Action Briefings and Related Materials*. London: Health Development Agency. http://www.publichealth.nice.org.uk/page.aspx?0=508114 (accessed 2 March 2006)

Kelly, M.P., Speller, V. and Meyrick, J. (2004b) *Getting Evidence into Practice in Public Health*. London: Health Development Agency. http:// www.publichealth.nice.org.uk/page.aspx?0=508124 (2 March 2006).

Kent, G. (2000a) Ethical principles, in D. Burton (ed.) *Research Training for Social Scientists*. London: Sage.

Kent, G. (2000b) Informed consent, in D. Burton (ed.) *Research Training for Social Scientists*. London: Sage.

Kirby, P. (2004) *A Guide to Actively Involving Young People in Research: For Researchers, Research Commissioners, and Managers*. Eastleigh: INVOLVE Support Unit.

Krieger, J., Allen, C., Cheadle, A., *et al.* (2002) Using community-based participatory research to address social determinants of health: lessons learnt from Seattle Partners for Healthy Communities, *Health Education and Behavior*, 29(3): 361–82.

Krueger, R.A. and King, J.A. (1998) *Involving Community Members in Focus Groups. Focus Group Kit 5*. London: Sage.

Labonte, R., Feather, J. and Hills, M. (1999) A story/dialogue method for health promotion knowledge development and evaluation, *Health Education Research*, 14(1): 39–50.

Laurance, J. (1998) Experts' 10 steps to health equality, *The Independent*, 12 November: 14

Lazenbatt, A., Orr, J., Bradley, M., McWhirter, L. and Chambers, M. (2000) Tackling inequalities in health and social wellbeing: evidence of 'good practice' by nurses, midwives and health visitors, *International Journal of Nursing Practice*, 6: 76–88.

Learmonth, A. and Mackie, P. (2000) Evaluating effectiveness in health promotion: a case of re-inventing the millstone? *Health Education Journal*, 59: 267–80.

Lee, R.M. (1993) *Doing Research on Sensitive Topics*. London: Sage.

Lever, M. and Moore, J. (2004) Experience in health promotion with community participation, *Community Practitioner*, 77(7): 261–4.

Lewis, J. (2001) Reflections on Evaluation in Practice, *Evaluation*, 7(3): 387–94.

Lewis, S.D., Johnson, V.R., Farris, R.P. and Will, J.C. (2004) Using success stories to share knowledge and lessons learned in health promotion, *Journal of Women's Health*, 13(5): 616–24.

LoBiondo-Wood, G. and Haber, J. (1994) *Nursing Research: Methods, Critical Appraisal, and Utilization*, 3rd edn. St. Louis, MO: Mosby.

London Health Observatory (2003) *Health Inequalities – Basket of Indicators*, http:// www.lho.org.uk/HEALTH_INEQUALITIES/BasketOfIndicators.aspx (accessed 30 October 2005).

Macaulay, A., Commanda, L., Freeman, W., *et al.* (1999) Participatory research maximises community and lay involvement, *British Medical Journal*, 319: 774–8.

MacDonald, G. (1996) Where next for evaluation? *Health Promotion International*, 11(3): 171–3.

Mackenzie, M. and Blamey, A. (2005) The practice and the theory: lessons from the application of a theories of change approach, *Evaluation*, 11(2): 151–68.

Mackenzie, M., Lawson, L. and Mackinnon, J. (2002) Generating learning, in L. Bauld and K. Judge (eds) *Learning from Health Action Zones*. Chichester: Aeneas Press.

MacPherson, K., Lattin-Rawstrone, R., Senior, R. and Barnes, J. (2005) Obstacles to gaining ethical approval from a multi-centre study of family support, *Children and Society*, 19: 237–45.

MacQueen, K.M. and Buehler, J.W. (2004) Ethics, practice and research in public health, *Amercian Journal of Public Health*, 94(6): 928–31.

Mager, R.F. (1975) *Preparing Instructional Objectives*. Belmont, CA: Fearon.

Markwell, S. (2003) *Partnership Working. A Consumer Guide to Resources*. London: Health Development Agency.

Markwell, S., Watson, J., Speller, V., Platt, S. and Younger, T. (2003) *The Working Partnership*. London: Health Development Agency.

McGuire, W.J. (1981) Theoretical foundations of campaigns, in R.E. Rice and W.J. Paisley (eds) *Public Communication Campaigns*. Beverly Hills, CA: Sage.

McKie, L., Barlow, J. and Gaunt-Richardson, P. (2002) *The Evaluation Journey. An Evaluation Resource for Community Groups*. Edinburgh: Action on Smoking and Health Scotland. http://www.ashscotland.org.uk/ash/ ash_display.jsp?pContentID=3367&p_applic=CCC&p_service=Content.show&# evaluationjourney (accessed 21 January 2006).

McLean, C.A. and Campbell, C.M. (2003) Locating research informants in a multi-ethnic community: ethnic identities, social networks and recruitment methods, *Ethnicity and Health*, 8(1): 41–61.

McNeish, D. and Downie, A. (n.d.) *Evaluation Toolkit: A Practical Guide to Project Evaluation*. Leeds: Leeds Health Action Zone and Barnardo's.

Meadows, P. (n.d.) *Guidance for Sure Start Local Evaluators and Programme Managers on the Estimation of Cost Effectiveness at a Local Level*. National Evaluation of Sure Start. http://www.ness.bbk.ac.uk/documents/GuidanceReports/167.pdf (accessed 14 March 2006).

Meulenberg-Buskens, I. (1996) Critical awareness in participatory research: an approach towards teaching and learning, in K. De Koning and M. Martin (eds) *Participatory Research in Health. Issues and Experiences*. London: Zed Books.

Meyrick, J. and Sinkler, P. (1999) *An Evaluation Resource for Healthy Living Centres*. London: Health Education Authority.

Milburn, K., Fraser, E., Secker, J. and Pavis, S. (1995) Combining methods in health promotion research: some considerations about appropriate use, *Health Education Journal*, 54: 347–56.

Miller, P. (2001) *Introduction to Health Economic Evaluation*. Trent Focus. http:// courses.essex.ac.uk/hs/hs915/Health%20Economic%20Evaluation.pdf (accessed 19 September 2005).

Milstein, R.L. and Wetterhall, S.F. (1999) Framework for program evaluation in public health. *MMWR Recommendations and Reports*, 48(11): 1–40. http://www.cdc.gov/ mmwr/preview/mmwrhtml/rr4811a1.htm (accessed 6 October 2005).

Minkler, M. (2004) Ethical challenges for the 'outside' researcher in community-based participatory research, *Health Education and Behavior*, 31(6): 684–7.

Moewaka Barnes, H. (2000) Collaboration in community action: a successful partnership between indigenous communities and researchers, *Health Promotion International*, 15(1): 17–25.

Moher, D., Schulz, K.F. and Altman, D.G. (2001) *Consort Statement*. Consort Group http://www.consort-statement.org/Statement/revisedstatement.htm (accessed 14 March 2005).

Murray, L. (2003) *Undercover in Sheffield. A Young People's Sexual Health Service Evaluation Scheme. Phase IR*. Sheffield: Centre for HIV and Sexual Health, South East Sheffield NHS Primary Care Trust, Sheffield Teenage Pregnancy Strategy.

Myers, P., Barnes, J. and Shemilt, I. (2004) *Using Existing Data in Sure Start Local Evaluations*. National Evaluation of Sure Start. http://www.ness.bbk.ac.uk/documents/GuidanceReports/395.pdf (accessed 14 March 2006).

Nancholas, S. (1998) How to do (or not to do) . . . a logical framework, *Health Policy and Planning*, 13(2): 189–93.

National Institute for Clinical Excellence (2005) *Nicotine Replacement Therapy (NRT) and Bupropion for Smoking Cessation*. Technology Appraisal Guidance No. 38, NICE. http://www.nice.org.uk/page.aspx?o=30631 (accessed 19 September 2005).

Neighbourhood Renewal Unit (2004) *English Indices of Deprivation 2004: Summary (Revised)*. Office of the Deputy Prime Minister. http://www.odpm.gov.uk/index.asp?id=1128442 (accessed 7 January 2006).

NESS Team (2005) *Early Impacts of Sure Start Local Programmes on Children and Families: Report 13*. London: DfES. www.surestart.gov.uk/_doc/P0001867.pdf (accessed 27 February 2006).

Newburn, T. (2001) What do we mean by evaluation? *Children and Society*, 15(1): 5–13.

Newell, C., South, J. and Green, J. (2004) *Sure Start Mellow Valley. Baseline User Satisfaction Survey*. Leeds: Centre for Health Promotion Research, Leeds Metropolitan University.

Nguyet Nguyen, M. and Otis, J. (2003) Evaluating the Fabreville Heart Health Program in Laval, Canada: a dialogue between the two paradigms, positivism and constructivism, *Health Promotion International*, 18(2): 127–34.

NHS Centre for Reviews and Dissemination (1999) Getting evidence into practice, *Effective Health Care*, 5(1).

NHS Research and Development Forum (2005) *Guidance on Developing Procedures within NHS Organisations for Appropriate Authorisation and Management of Research and Related Projects*. http://www.rdforum.nhs.uk/docs/categorising_projects_guidance.doc (accessed 21 January 2006).

Nutbeam, D. (1998) Evaluating health promotion – progress, problems and solutions, *Health Promotion International*, 13(1): 27–43.

Nutbeam, D., Smith, C., Murphy, S. and Catford, J. (1993) Maintaining evaluation designs in long term community based health promotion programmes: Heartbeat Wales case study, *Journal of Epidemiology and Community Health*, 47: 127–33.

Oakley, A. (1998a) Experimentation and social interventions: a forgotten but important history, *British Medical Journal*, 317(7167): 1239–42.

Oakley, A. (1998b) Experimentation in social science: the case of health promotion, *Social Sciences in Health*, 4(2): 73–89.

Oakley, A., Strange, V., Toroyan, T., *et al*. (2003) Using random allocation to evaluate social interventions: three recent UK examples, *Annals of American Academy of Political and Social Science*, 589: 170–89.

Oldenburg, B.F., Sallis, J.F., French, M.L. and Owen, N. (1999) Health promotion research and the diffusion and institutionalization of interventions, *Health Education Research*, 14(1): 121–30.

Oliver, P. (2003) *The Student's Guide to Research Ethics*. Maidenhead: Open University Press.

Ontario Clearing House (n.d.) *Build Communities: Using Stories in Health Promotion*.

http://www.opc.on.ca/english/our_programs/hlth_promo/resources/stories/using_
stories.htm (accessed 25 November 2005).

Øvretveit, J. (1998) *Evaluating Health Interventions*. Buckingham: Open University Press.

Oxfam (1999) Measuring women's empowerment in India, *Links* (July).

Packham, C. (1998) Community auditing as community development, *Community Development Journal*, 33(3): 249–59.

Parlett, M. and Hamilton, D. (1972) *Evaluation as Illumination: A New Approach to the Study of Innovatory Programmes*, Occasional Paper No. 9. Edinburgh: Centre for Research in the Educational Sciences, University of Edinburgh.

Parry, O., Gnich, W. and Platt, S. (2001) Principles in practice: reflections on a 'postpositivist' approach to evaluation research, *Health Education Research*, 16(2): 215–26.

Parry-Langdon, N., Bloor, M., Audrey, S. and Holliday, J. (2003) Process evaluation of health promotion interventions, *Policy and Politics*, 31(2): 207–16.

Patton, M.Q. (1987) *How to Use Qualitative Methods in Evaluation*. London: Sage.

Patton, M.Q. (1997) *Utilisation Focused Evaluation*. Thousand Oaks, CA: Sage.

Pawson, R. (2002) Evidence-based policy: the promise of 'realist synthesis', *Evaluation*, 8(3): 340–58.

Pawson, R. and Myhill, A. (2001) *Learning Lessons: Enhancing Evaluation through Research Review*, TRL Report 507. Crowthorne: TRL Limited.

Pawson, R. and Tilley, N. (1997) *Realistic Evaluation*. London: Sage.

Perkins, E.R., Simnett, I. and Wright, L. (1999) *Evidence-Based Health Promotion*. Chichester: Wiley.

Petersen, A. and Lupton, D. (1996) *The New Public Health: Health and Self in the Age of Risk*. London: Sage.

Phillips, C., Palfrey, C. and Thomas, P. (1994) *Evaluating Health and Social Care*. London: Macmillan.

Pollitt, C. (1999) Stunted by stakeholders? Limits to collaborative evaluation, *Public Policy and Administration*, 14(2): 77–90.

Potvin, L. and Richard, L. (2001) Evaluating community health promotion programmes, in I. Rootman, M.S. Goodstadt, B. Hyndman, D.V. McQueen, L. Potvin, J. Springett and E. Ziglio (eds) *Evaluation in Health Promotion. Principles and Perspectives*. Copenhagen: WHO Europe.

Potvin, L., Haddad, S. and Frohlich, K.L. (2001) Beyond process and outcome: a comprehensive approach to evaluating health promotion programmes, in I. Rootman, M.S. Goodstadt, B. Hyndman, D.V. McQueen, L. Potvin, J. Springett and E. Ziglio (eds) *Evaluation in Health Promotion. Principles and Perspectives*. Copenhagen: WHO Europe.

Pridmore, P. (1996) Visualising health: exploring perceptions of children using the draw and write method, *Promotion & Education*, 3(4): 11–15.

Punch, K.F. (2005) *Introduction to Social Research*, 2nd edn. London: Sage.

Raphael, D. (2000) The question of evidence in health promotion, *Health Promotion International*, 15(4): 355–67.

RE-AIM (2004) *Applying the RE-AIM Framework to Health Behavior Interventions: How Well Does Research Translate into Practice?* http://www.re-aim.org/2003/researches/defined_res.html (accessed 16 March 2006).

Rifkin, S.B., Muller, F. and Bichmann, W. (1988) Primary health care: on measuring participation, *Social Science and Medicine*, 26(9): 931–40.

Rifkin, S.B., Lewando-Hundt, G. and Draper, A.K. (2000) *Participatory Approaches in Health Promotion and Health Planning. A Literature Review*. London: Health Development Agency.

Riley, C. and Riley, J. (1998) Outcome indicators: friends or enemies? *Managing Community Care*, 6(6): 246–53.

Riley, T. and Hawe, P. (2005) Researching practice: the methodological case for narrative enquiry, *Health Education Research*, 20(2): 226–36.

Roberts, M. and Roche, M. (n.d.) *Quantifying Social Capital: Measuring the Intangible in the Local Policy Context*. http://www.radstats.org.uk/no076/robertsandroche.htm (accessed 31 October 2005).

Rodmell, S. and Watt, A. (1986) *The Politics of Health Education: Raising the Issues*. London: Routledge & Kegan Paul.

Rogers, E.M. (1995) *The Diffusion of Innovations*. 4th edn. New York: Free Press.

Rogers, E.M. and Shoemaker, F.F. (1971) *Communication of Innovations*. New York: Free Press.

Rootman, I., Goodstadt, M.S., Potvin, L. and Springett, J. (2001) A framework for health promotion evaluation, in I. Rootman, M.S. Goodstadt, B. Hyndman, D.V. McQueen, L. Potvin, J. Springett and E. Ziglio (eds) *Evaluation in Health Promotion. Principles and Perspectives*. Denmark: WHO Europe.

Ross, S., Lavis, J., Roderiguez, C., Woodside, J. and Denis, J.L. (2003) Partnership experiences: involving decision-makers in the research process, *Journal of Health Services Research and Policy*, 8(Suppl. 2): 26–34.

Royle, J., Steel, R., Hanley, B. and Bradburn, J. (2001) *Getting Involved in Research: A Guide for Consumers*. Eastleigh: Consumers in NHS Research Support Unit.

Ryan, W. (1976) *Blaming the Victim*. New York: Vintage Books.

Rychetnik, L. and Wise, M. (2004) Advocating evidence-based health promotion: reflections and a way forward, *Health Promotion International*, 19(2): 247–57.

Sackett, D.L., Rosenberg, W.M.C., Gray, J.A.M., Haynes, R.B. and Richardson, W.S. (1996) Evidence based medicine: what it is and what it isn't, *British Medical Journal*, 312: 71–2.

St Leger, A.S., Schnieden, H. and Walsworth-Bell, J.P. (1992) *Evaluating Health Services' Effectiveness: A Guide for Health Professionals, Service Managers and Policy Makers*. Milton Keynes: Open University Press.

Salvin, J. (2004) Qualitative research of young males' use of a teenage health bus. MSc dissertation, Leeds Metropolitan University.

Sanderson, I. (2000) Evaluation in complex policy systems, *Evaluation*, 6(4): 433–54.

Scott, D. (1998) Qualitative approaches to evaluations of health-promoting activities, in D. Scott and R. Weston (eds) *Evaluating Health Promotion*. Cheltenham: Stanley Thornes.

Sentinella, J. (2004) *Guidelines for Evaluating Road Safety Education Interventions*. London: Department for Transport.

Shea, S. and Basch, C.E. (1990) A review of five major community-based cardiovascular disease prevention programs. Part 1: Rationale, design and theoretical framework, *American Journal of Health Promotion*, 4(3): 203–13.

Shengelia, B., Tandon, A., Adams, O.B. and Murray, C.J.L. (2005) Access, utilization, quality and effective coverage: an integrated conceptual framework and measurement strategy, *Social Science and Medicine*, 61: 97–109.

Silverman, D. (1985) *Qualitative Methodology and Sociology*. Aldershot: Gower.

Simpson, E.L. and House, A.O. (2002) Involving users in the delivery and evaluation of mental health services: systematic review, *British Medical Journal*, 325: 1265–9.

Smith, H.W. (1975) *Strategies of Social Research: The Methodological Imagination*. London: Prentice Hall.

Smithies, J. and Adams, L. (1993) Walking the tightrope. Issues in evaluation and community participation for Health for All, in J. Davies and M. Kelly (eds) *Healthy Cities: Research and Practice*. London: Routledge.

Social Exclusion Unit (2001) *Preventing Social Exclusion*. London: Cabinet Office.

Social Research Association (2003) *Ethical Guidelines*. http://www.the-sra.org.uk/ethicals.htm (accessed 25 January 2006).

South, J. (2004) Rising to the challenge: a study of patient and public involvement in four Primary Care Trusts, *Primary Health Care Research and Development*, 5(2): 125–34.

South, J. and Green, E. (2001) Learning from practice: evaluating a community involvement team within a Health Action Zone., *Research, Policy and Planning*, 19(3): 1–9.

South, J. and Tilford, S. (2000) Perceptions of research and evaluation in health promotion practice and influences on activity, *Health Education Research*, 15(6): 729–41.

South, J., Fairfax, P. and Green, E. (2005) Developing an assessment tool for evaluating community involvement, *Health Expectations*, 8: 64–73.

Speller, V., Learmonth, A. and Harrison, D. (1997) The search for evidence of effective health promotion, *British Medical Journal*, 315: 361–3.

Springett, J. (1998a) *Practical Guidance on Evaluating Health Promotion*. Copenhagen: WHO Europe.

Springett, J. (1998b) Quality measures and evaluation of Healthy City policy initiatives, in J.K. Davies and G. Macdonald (eds) *Quality, Evidence and Effectiveness in Health Promotion*. London: Routledge.

Springett, J. (2001a) Appropriate approaches to the evaluation of health promotion, *Critical Public Health*, 11(2): 139–51.

Springett, J. (2001b) Participatory approaches to evaluation in health promotion, in I. Rootman, M.S Goodstadt, B. Hyndman, D.V. McQueen, L. Potvin, J. Springett and E. Ziglio (eds) *Evaluation in Health Promotion. Principles and Perspectives*. Copenhagen: WHO Europe.

Springett, J. and Young, A. (2002) Evaluating community-level projects: comparing theories of change and participatory approaches, in L. Bauld and K. Judge (eds) *Learning from Health Action Zones*. Chichester: Aeneas Press.

Stephenson, J. and Imrie, J. (1998) Why do we need randomised controlled trials to assess behavioural interventions? *British Medical Journal*, 316: 611–13.

Suchman, E.A. (1967) *Evaluative Research: Principles in Public Service and Action Programs*. New York: Russell Sage.

Sullivan, H., Barnes, M. and Matka, E. (2002) Building collaborative capacity through 'theories of change', *Evaluation*, 8(2): 205–26.

Sullivan, M., Kone, A., Senturia, K.D., *et al.* (2001) Researcher and researched – community perspectives: toward bridging the gap, *Health Education and Behavior*, 28(2): 130–49.

Swann, C., Falce, C., Morgan, A., Kelly, M., Powel, G., Carmona, C., Taylor, L. and Taske, N. (2005) *HDA Evidence Base Process and Quality Standards Manual for Evidence Briefings*, 3rd edn. London: Health Development Agency.

Swords, M. (2002) *Built-on, Not Bolt-on: Engaging Young People in Evaluation*. New Opportunities Fund. http://www.nof.org.uk/documents/live/2665p_Engaging_young_people_report.pdf (accessed 21 January 2006).

Tandon, R. (1996) The historical roots and contemporary tendencies in participatory research: implications for health care, in K. De Koning and M. Martin (eds) *Participatory Research in Health. Issues and Experiences*. London: Zed Books.

Tesh, S. (1988) *Hidden Arguments*. New Brunswick, NJ: Rutgers University Press.

Thompson, J.C. (1992) Progam evaluation within a health promotion framework, *Canadian Journal of Public Health*, 83(Suppl. 1): S67– S71.

Thurston, W.E. and Potvin, L. (2003) Evaluability assessment: a tool for incorporating evaluation in social change programmes, *Evaluation*, 9(4): 453–69.

Thurston, W.E., Vollman, A.R. and Burgess, M.M. (2003) Ethical review of health promotion program evaluation proposals, *Health Promotion Practice*, 4(1): 45–50.

Tilford, S., Green, J. and Tones, K. (2003) *Values, Health Promotion and Public Health*. Leeds, Centre for Health Promotion Research, Leeds Metropolitan University.

Tod, A.M., Nicholson, P. and Allmark, P. (2002) Ethical review of health service research in the UK: implications for nursing, *Journal of Advanced Nursing*, 40(4): 379–86.

Tolley, E.E. and Bentley, M.E. (1996) Training issues for the use of participatory research methods in health, in K. De Koning and M. Martin (eds) *Participatory Research in Health. Issues and Experiences*. London: Zed Books.

Tolley, K. (1993) *Health Promotion: How to Measure Cost-Effectiveness*. London: Health Education Authority.

Tolley, K., Buck, D. and Godfrey, C. (1996) Health promotion and health economics, *Health Education Research*, 11(3): 361–4.

Tones, K. (1997) Beyond the randomised controlled trial: a case for 'judicial review', *Health Education Research*, 12(2): i–iv.

Tones, K. (1998) Effectiveness in health promotion: indicators and evidence of success, in D. Scott and R. Weston (eds) *Evaluating Health Promotion*. Cheltenham: Stanley Thornes.

Tones, K. and Green, J. (2004) *Health Promotion. Planning and Strategies*. London: Sage.

Tones, K. and Tilford, S. (1994) *Health Education: Effectiveness, Efficiency and Equity*, 2nd edn. London: Chapman & Hall.

Tones, K. and Tilford, S. (2001) *Health Promotion: Effectiveness, Efficiency and Equity*, 3rd edn. Cheltenham: Nelson Thornes.

Townend, D.M.R. (2000) How does substantive law currently regulate social science research? in D. Burton (ed.) *Research Training for Social Scientists*. London: Sage.

Trickett, E. (1998) Toward a framework for defining and resolving ethical issues in the protection of communities involved in primary prevention projects, *Ethics and Behaviour*, 8: 321–37.

Truman, C. and Raine, P. (2001) Involving users in evaluation: the social relations of user participation in health research, *Critical Public Health*, 11(3): 215–29.

Truman, C., Mertens, D.M. and Humphris, B. (eds) (2000) *Research and Inequality*. London: Routledge.

UK Evaluation Society (2003a) *Glossary of Evaluation Terms*. http:// www.evaluation.org.uk/Pub_library/Glossary.htm (accessed 27 May 2005).

UK Evaluation Society (2003b) *UK Evaluation Society Good Practice Guidelines*. http:// evaluation.org.uk/Pub_library/Good_Practice.htm (accessed 21 January 2006).

University of Kansas (n.d.) *Community Tool Box. Part J. Evaluating Community Programs and Initiatives*. http://ctb.ku.edu/tools/en/tools_toc.htm#partJ (accessed 21 January 2006).

Waa, A., Holibar, F. and Spinola, C. (1998) *Planning and Doing Programme Evaluation: An Introductory Guide for Health Promotion*. Auckland: Alcohol and Public Health Research Unit, University of Auckland. http://www.aphru.ac.nz/services/services/ manual.htm (accessed 21 January 2006).

Wadsworth, Y., Wierenga, A. and Wilson, G. (2004) *Writing Narrative Action Evaluation Reports in Health Promotion – Guidelines, Resource Kit and Case Studies*. Melbourne: Department of Human Services, State Government of Victoria. http://

www.health.vic.gov.au/healthpromotion/hp_practice/eval_dissem.htm#narrative (accessed 1 December 2005).

Walden, V. and Baxter, D. (2001) The comprehensive approach: an evaluation model to assess HIV/AIDS-related behaviour change in developing countries, *Evaluation*, 7(4): 439–52.

Wallerstein, N. (1999) Power between evaluator and community: research relationships within New Mexico's healthier communities, *Social Science and Medicine*, 49: 39–53.

Wallerstein, N. and Bernstein, E. (1994) Introduction to community empowerment, participatory education and health, *Health Education Quarterly*, 21(2): 141–8.

Walter, I., Davies, H. and Nutley, S. (2003) Increasing research impact through partnerships: evidence from outside health care, *Journal of Health Services Research and Policy*, 8(Suppl. 2): 58–61.

Wang, G. and Macera, C.A. (2005) A cost–benefit analysis of physical activity using bike/pedestrian trails, *Health Promotion Practice*, 6(2): 174–9.

Wanless, D. (2002) *Securing Our Future Health: Taking a Long-Term View*. HM Treasury. http://www.hm-treasury.gov.uk/Consultations_and_Legislation/wanless/con-sult_wanless_final.cfm (accessed 30 July 2002).

Watson, B. and Scraton, S. (2001) Confronting whiteness? Researching the leisure lives of South Asian mothers, *Journal of Gender Studies*, 10(3): 265–77.

Weiss, C.H. (1972) *Evaluation Research: Methods of Assessing Program Effectiveness*. Englewood Cliffs, NJ: Prentice Hall.

Wellings, K. and MacDowall, W. (2000) Evaluating mass media approaches to health promotion: a review of methods, *Health Education*, 100(1): 23–32.

White, A. and Cash, K. (2005) *Report on the First Phase of the Study on Men's Usage of the Bradford Health of Men Services*. Leeds: Leeds Metropolitan University.

Whitehead, M. (1993) The ownership of research, in J. Davies and M. Kelly (eds) *Healthy Cities: Research and Practice*. London: Routledge.

WHO Europe Working Group on Health Promotion Evaluation (1998) *Health Promotion Evaluation: Recommendations to Policy Makers*. Brighton: WHO Europe.

WHO Regional Office for Europe (1991) *Community Involvement in Health: Indicators*, EUR/ICP/PHC335. Copenhagen: WHO Regional Office for Europe.

WHO Regional Office for Europe (2002) *Community Participation in Local Health and Sustainable Development. Approaches and Techniques*, European Sustainable Development and Health Series No. 4, EUR/ICP/POLC 06 03 05D. Copenhagen: WHO Regional Office for Europe.

Wiggers, J. and Sanson-Fisher, R. (1998) Evidence-based health promotion, in R. Scott and R. Weston (eds) *Evaluation Health Promotion*. Cheltenham: Stanley Thornes.

Wilcox, D. (1994) *The Guide to Effective Participation*. Brighton: Partnership Books.

Williams, G. and Popay, J. (1994) Researching the people's health. Dilemmas and opportunities for social scientists, in J. Popay and G. Williams (eds) *Researching the People's Health*. London: Routledge.

Williams, R. and Wright, J. (1998) Epidemiological issues in health needs assessment, *British Medical Journal*, 316: 1379–82.

Wimbush, E. and Watson, J. (2000) An evaluation framework for health promotion: theory, quality and effectiveness, *Evaluation*, 6(3): 301–21.

Witkin, S.L. (2000) An integrative human rights approach to social research, in C. Truman, D.M. Mertens and B. Humphries (eds) *Research and Inequality*. London: Routledge.

Woolf, F. (1999) *Partnerships for Learning. A Guide to Evaluating Arts Education Projects*. London: Arts Council for England.

Woolf, F. (2004) *Partnerships for Learning. A Guide to Evaluating Arts Education Projects*.

London: Arts Council. http://www.artscouncil.org.uk/documents/publications/phpLYOOMa.pdf (accessed 22 January 2006).

World Bank (2004) *Monitoring & Evaluation: Some Tools, Methods & Approaches*. http://lnweb18.worldbank.org/oed/oeddoclib.nsf/DocUNIDViewForJavaSearch/A5EF-BB5D776B67D285256B1E0079C9A3/$file/MandE_tools_methods_approaches.pdf (accessed 21 January 2006).

World Health Organization (1986) *Ottawa Charter for Health Promotion*. International Conference on Health Promotion, Ottawa, 17–21 November. Copenhagen: WHO Regional Office for Europe.

World Health Organization (1998) *Health Promotion Evaluation: Recommendations to Policymakers: Report of the WHO European Working Group on Health Promotion Evaluation*. Copenhagen: WHO Regional Office for Europe.

World Medical Association (2004) *World Medical Association Declaration of Helsinki*. http://www.wma.net/e/policy/b3.htm (accessed 11 July 2005).

Worthen, B.R., Sanders, J.R. and Fitzpatrick, J.L. (1996) *Program Evaluation: Alternative Approaches and Practical Guidelines*, 2nd edn. New York: Longman, Inc.

Wright, L. (1999) Evaluation in health promotion: the proof of the pudding? in E. Perkins, I. Simnett and L. Wright (eds). *Evidence Based Health Promotion*. England: Wiley.

Wulf, K.N. (1993) A study of the implementation of the DARE programme in law enforcement agencies. Paper presented to the Crime Prevention Advisory Council, University of Southern California, Los Angeles.

Yorkshire Forward (2000) *Active Partners. Benchmarking Community Participation in Regeneration*. Leeds: Yorkshire Forward.

Index

Related books from Open University Press

Purchase from www.openup.co.uk or order through your local bookseller

UNDERSTANDING PUBLIC HEALTH SERIES

Edited by Nick Black and Rosalind Raine

There is an increasing global awareness of the inevitable limits of individual health care and of the need to complement such services with effective public health strategies. Understanding Public Health is an innovative series of twenty books, published by Open University Press in collaboration with the London School of Hygiene & Tropical Medicine. It provides self-directed learning covering the major issues in public health affecting low, middle and high income countries.

The series is aimed at those studying public health, either by distance learning or more traditional methods, as well as public health practitioners and policy makers.

UNDERSTANDING HEALTH SERVICES

Nick Black and Reinhold Gruen

No single discipline can provide a full account of how and why health care is the way it is. This book provides you with a series of conceptual frameworks which help to unravel the apparent complexity that confronts the inexperienced observer. It demonstrates the need for contributions from medicine, sociology, economics, history and epidemiology. It also shows the necessity to consider health care at three key levels: individual patients and their experiences; health care organisations such as health centres and hospitals; and regional and national institutions such as governments and health insurance bodies.

The book examines:

- Inputs to health services
- Processes of care
- Outcomes
- Organization of services
- Improving the quality of health care

Contents

Overview of the book – Section 1: Introduction – A systems approach to health services – Challenges facing health services – Formal and lay care – Section 2: Inputs to health care – Diseases and medical knowledge – Medical paradigms – Staff: the challenge of professionalism – Funding health care – Section 3: Processes of health care – The need and demand for health care – The relationship between need and use – Staff-patient interactions – Public as consumers and policy makers – Section 4: Outcome of health care - Outcomes – Section 5: Organization of services – Analysing health systems – Why are health systems the way they are? – Low and middle income countries: from colonial inheritance to primary care – Low and middle income countries: from comprehensive primary care to global initiatives – Health services in high income countries – Section 6: Quality improvement - Defining good quality health services – Performance assessment – Improving quality of care – Glossary – Index.

256pp   0 335 21838 5 (Paperback)

UNDERSTANDING PUBLIC HEALTH SERIES

Edited by Nick Black and Rosalind Raine

There is an increasing global awareness of the inevitable limits of individual health care and of the need to complement such services with effective public health strategies. Understanding Public Health is an innovative series of twenty books, published by Open University Press in collaboration with the London School of Hygiene & Tropical Medicine. It provides self-directed learning covering the major issues in public health affecting low, middle and high income countries.

The series is aimed at those studying public health, either by distance learning or more traditional methods, as well as public health practitioners and policy makers.

MAKING HEALTH POLICY

Kent Buse, Nicolas Mays and Gill Walt

Surprisingly little guidance is available to public health practitioners who wish to understand how issues get onto policy agendas, how policy makers treat evidence and why some policy initiatives are implemented while others languish. This book views power and process as integral to understanding policy and focuses on the three key elements in policy making: the context, the actors and the processes. It is a guide for those who wish to improve their skills in navigating and managing the health policy process, irrespective of the health issue or setting.

The book examines:

*   Policy analysis
*   Power
*   Private and public sectors
*   Policy makers
*   Policy implementation
*   Research and policy

Contents

Overview of the book – The health policy framework: Context, process and actors – Power and the policy process – The state and private sector in health policy – Agenda setting – Government and the policy process – Interest groups and the policy process – Policy implementation – Globalizing the policy process – Research, evaluation and policy – Doing policy analysis – Glossary – Acronyms – Index.

216pp   0 335 21839 3 (Paperback)

UNDERSTANDING PUBLIC HEALTH SERIES

Edited by Nick Black and Rosalind Raine

There is an increasing global awareness of the inevitable limits of individual health care and of the need to complement such services with effective public health strategies. Understanding Public Health is an innovative series of twenty books, published by Open University Press in collaboration with the London School of Hygiene & Tropical Medicine. It provides self-directed learning covering the major issues in public health affecting low, middle and high income countries.

The series is aimed at those studying public health, either by distance learning or more traditional methods, as well as public health practitioners and policy makers.

ISSUES IN PUBLIC HEALTH

Joceline Pomerleau and Martin McKee (eds)

This book is for those who want to answer the question 'What is public health?'. Much of modern public health is about tackling strong vested interests head on, empowering people so they can make healthy decisions, and recognising the political nature of the issues. If a society is to achieve these things, it needs public health practitioners with the necessary knowledge, skills and vision.

This book looks at the foundation of public health, its historical evolution, the themes that underpin public health, the increasing importance of globalization and the most important causes of avoidable disease and injury.

These include:

- Transport
- Tobacco
- Nutrition
- Infectious disease
- Waste disposal

Contents
*Overview of the book – **Section 1: Foundation of modern public health** - The emergence of public health and the centrality of values – Data on populations and mortality – The burden of disease and other summary measures of population health – Inequalities in health – Impact of healthcare on population health – Assessing the impact on population health of policies in other sectors – **Section 2: Major determinants of health –** The changing nature of infectious disease – Tobacco: a public health emergency – Food, trade and health – Drains, dustbins and diseases – Glossary – Index.*

240pp   0 335 21836 9 (Paperback)

PUBLIC HEALTH FOR THE 21st CENTURY
NEW PERSPECTIVES ON POLICY, PARTICIPATION AND PRACTICE

Judy Orme, Jane Powell, Pat Taylor, Tony Harrison and Melanie Grey

This book explores the meaning of the 'new' public health within current debates, and the policy changes that are reshaping the context for public health. It moves away from public health medicine to a multi-disciplinary approach to public health concerns. This book asks:

- Why is a multidisciplinary approach to public health important and where is its future?
- What is the nature of the new multidisciplinary public health?
- How can multidisciplinary public health professionals move towards an evidence-informed public health practice?

With analysis and reflection upon public health history theories, research and practice, *Public Health for the 21st Century* engages advanced undergraduate and graduate students, trainees and professionals across a broad range of disciplines.

Contents

368pp   0 335 21193 3 (Paperback)   0 335 21194 1 (Hardback)

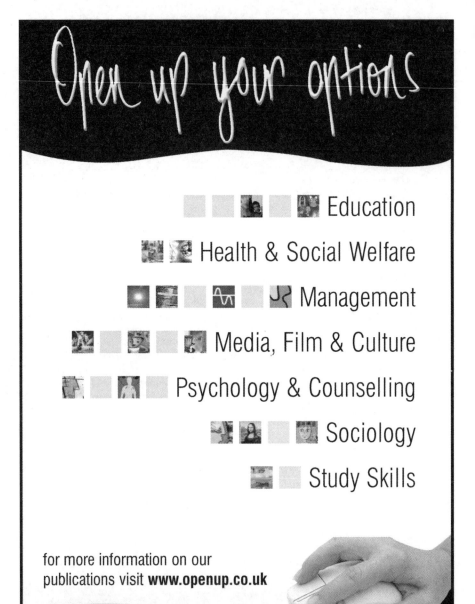

Open up your options

Education

Health & Social Welfare

Management

Media, Film & Culture

Psychology & Counselling

Sociology

Study Skills

for more information on our
publications visit **www.openup.co.uk**

OPEN UNIVERSITY PRESS
McGraw - Hill Education